# Lifetime Weight Control

## Seven Steps to Achieving and Maintaining a Healthy Weight

### Patrick Fanning

*Publisher's Note*

*This publication is designed to provide accurate and authoritative information in regard to the subject matter covered. It is sold with the understanding that the publisher is not engaged in rendering psychological, financial, legal, or other professional services. If expert assistance or counseling is needed, the services of a competent professional should be sought.*

# Table of Contents

# A

# How To Use This Book

This is not a diet book. I know you've read that claim before, but this time it's for real. This book has no calorie counting, no weighing yourself or your food, no measuring, no food restrictions, no portion control, and no weight loss goals.

This isn't even a weight loss book. It's a weight *control* or *stabilization* book. The idea is to help you arrive at a comfortable, healthy, acceptable weight that you can maintain, without dieting, for the rest of your life.

The seven steps taught to accomplish this are very simple:

1. Eat Spontaneously ... whatever you want, without dieting, because diets not only don't work, but are harmful and actually cause net weight gain.

2. Accept Yourself ... so that you can resist the cruel fallacies that excess weight is inherently ugly, shameful, and unhealthy.

3. Determine How and Why You Eat ... so that you can learn to eat only when you're really hungry, not because you're bored, sad, lonely, angry, or anxious.

4.  Satisfy Emotional Needs Directly ... instead of indirectly by eating.

5.  Improve Nutrition ... by eating for health instead of weight loss.

6.  Increase Activity ... for fun and health instead of weight loss.

7.  Stick With It ... year after year, with the help of proven cognitive behavioral techniques.

Abandoning diets and eating spontaneously may sound impossible, frightening, or crazy to you at this point. If so, you need to approach this idea slowly and cautiously. The next two chapters will explain the reasoning behind spontaneous eating and help you put any doubts and fears to rest. Read them carefully before you make a final judgment about whether spontaneous eating is for you.

Read this book slowly. Be prepared to reread some sections several times. The advice in this book is based on recent research that contradicts several traditional, common sense notions about weight and dieting. It will take you some time to absorb and understand the fine points.

Follow the instructions. Don't just "read through" the self-help exercises. Lifetime weight control is a skill, like driving a car, baking a pie, or singing a song. If you don't practice by doing the exercises, you won't learn the skill.

Gaining new skills takes time. Give the ideas and exercises in this book time to sink in. If you are a chronic dieter, it has probably taken you years to become as obsessed with food and your weight as you are. Give yourself at least a fraction of that time to change your life. If you have been dieting off and on for a several years, you should plan on taking at least two years to make lifetime weight control work for you.

This book is for both men and women. However, most of the people used as examples are women, and I often assume that the reader is a woman. This is intentional. In our culture, the problems surrounding weight control are much more severe for women. More women than men suffer from obsessions about weight and food, and their wounds run deeper. However, the solutions presented will work as well for men as for women.

This is a self-help book in an area where self-help is sometimes inappropriate or not enough. If any of these statements apply to you you should seek professional help from an eating disorder specialist such as a medical doctor or a psychologist:

> You are very underweight.
> You regularly make yourself throw up.
> You take a lot of laxatives or diuretics.
> You are extremely depressed or anxious.

If you decide to get weight control help from a therapist or M.D., be careful. Find one who understands that dieting is ultimately useless. Find one who will do more than assist you to lose weight on yet another diet. Find one who will support your efforts to rid yourself once and for all of your obsession with weight.

Finally, congratulations on starting this book. You are about to embark on a challenging but exciting adventure: becoming a fit, healthy person who enjoys all kinds of food freely and effortlessly maintains a stable weight without obsessing about food.

# B

# The Dieting Nightmare

Did you ever have a helpless nightmare? You know the kind: you're desperately looking for something that eludes you. You're naked and everyone can see you but you can't seem to get your clothes on. You're late for school but you can't get out of the house. A man with a knife is chasing you and you can't move. Your child is about to fall out a window and you need to cry out a warning but your throat's frozen shut.

If you've had one of these dreams, you know how vivid and utterly convincing they can be and what a relief it is to wake up and realize that it was all just a dream.

I want this book to be like waking from a nightmare for you—waking from the nightmare of chronic dieting.

Chronic dieting is a living nightmare. You're desperately seeking a weight or shape that eludes you. Everyone can see how fat you are and you can't cover it up. You know you should eat less and exercise more but you can't seem to put it together consistently. Overwhelming cravings stab you like a knife in your stomach. Sometimes you feel so depressed or afraid of losing control that you could just cry.

You can wake up from this nightmare. You can feel the blessed relief of realizing that it was all a dream. You can take the first step toward lifetime weight control. You can stop dieting and just eat what you want.

That's right. You can stop dieting and eat spontaneously. You *should* stop dieting. You *must* stop dieting. I mean exactly what I'm saying. The first step of lifetime weight control really is to stop all forms of dieting and just learn to enjoy food again. It's a simple step, but very hard to make. Simple because you don't have to *do* anything, just *stop* doing something. Hard because it flies in the face of accepted wisdom. It's like someone told you, "Well, it was all a mistake. The world isn't round after all. It's a cube."

Eating whatever you want, without any thought about calories or fat, is such a strange and scary idea that I'm going to approach it very slowly and cautiously. Don't make any changes in your diet or eating patterns right now. Just continue what you're doing, reserve judgment, and keep reading. You may be tempted to look further in the book to see what's coming: self-acceptance, why and how you eat, satisfying emotional needs directly, improving nutrition, increasing activity, and so on. It's fine to look ahead. Just don't try to put any of the later steps into action until you have read and absorbed this chapter and the next chapter.

This chapter and the next one lay the groundwork for the all-important first step of learning to eat spontaneously again. In this chapter I'll point out the harm dieting can do both to your body and your self-esteem, and share some reasons why dieting doesn't work. In the next chapter you'll learn how to handle the very real fears that can overtake you when you seriously consider giving up dieting.

Again, please read this chapter and the next one carefully before attempting to take the first step of eating spontaneously.

## Dieting Is Harmful

If you get only one thing from this book, get this: that dieting is harmful. It burns out your body, clouds your mind, inflames your feelings, erodes your self-esteem, saps your energy, poisons your pleasures, perverts your appetite, strains your relationships, and shortens your life. And for what? Short-term weight loss and long-term *nothing*.

I have a friend named Janice who considers herself to be about twenty pounds overweight right now. Actually, she looks fine to me, but she'd really like to "drop twenty pounds." And she can do it any time she wants because she's had lots of practice. Over the five years I've known her, Janice has lost 160 pounds!

As much as I love Janice, I hope she doesn't go back on a diet. When she's dieting, she's hell to live with. She gets grouchy and depressed. If I invite her over for dinner, she probably wont' come, even if I offer to let her pick the menu. Eating just isn't any fun for her when she's dieting. When she does visit, all she can talk about is calories and carbohydrates and what she'd really like to eat if she could have any-thing she wanted. Her natural sparkle and humor is dampened when she's dieting. She doesn't have any energy or enthusiasm. Frankly, it's boring to be around Janice when she's dieting, and it's sad to watch her.

It's sad because Janice is *not* one of those seriously overweight people who save their own lives by going from 320 pounds down to 160. Hers is a much more common case. She weighed the same five years as she weighs now. She lost her 160 pounds in five years by losing (and regaining) *the same twenty pounds* eight times over! She put herself through eight different diets and did incalculable damage to her health and her self-esteem, all for nothing.

### Eating Disorders

*Question:* What is the most common eating disorder in the United States?
*Answer: Chronic dieting.*

Not anorexia nervosa. Not bulimia. Those two are the answers that spring to mind, but chronic dieting affects more people and causes more physical and mental suffering than anorexia and bulimia combined.

How can you tell if you have a chronic dieting "eating disorder?" Check the list of symptoms below. If most of them apply to you, you are suffering from chronic dieting, even if you are not officially on a diet right now.

I desperately want to be thin.
I am preoccupied with eating less.
I feel frequent hunger pangs and cravings.
I immediately notice fatness or thinness of others.
I always notice my own fatness or thinness.
I see myself as fatter than I actually am.
I hate myself when I eat something "bad."

I am afraid of losing control and gaining weight.
I exercise like crazy or think I should.
I often feel depressed and/or lonely.
I have stopped having periods.
I have occasional binges where I can't stop eating or can't get full.

These symptoms of chronic dieting can also be symptoms of the less common, more serious eating disorders of anorexia nervosa and bulimia. It's more a difference in degree than a difference in kind.

If you have *all* of these symptoms with the exception of binging and you have lost 20 percent or more of your original weight, then you have probably crossed over the line into full-fledged anorexia nervosa. You should see a therapist right away. You're endangering your health and maybe your life.

If you have almost all of these symptoms and you also try to purge yourself by vomiting, laxatives, or diuretics, then you probably are suffering from bulimia—even if you haven't lost a lot of weight. You too should see a therapist before you damage your health further.

### How Dieting Harms You

First of all, dieting harms your body. When you haven't been getting enough food for a period of time, your metabolism and your pulse rate slow down. You may feel dizzy, listless, and without energy. You lose not only reserves of fat but also muscle tissue, so you are weaker. When you regain weight after dieting, you gain back the fat but not the muscle, so losing weight by dieting and gaining it back makes you less fit. Dieting decreases your sex drive and can make some women's periods stop entirely. Dieting causes intense cravings for food. When you satisfy those cravings, you are likely to binge and eat too much, putting another kind of strain on your body.

Repeated dieting usually sets up a cycle of weight loss and gain. This weight fluctuation puts a strain on your body that is worse than the strain of just staying at a stable, relatively high weight.

Besides hurting your body, dieting also hurts you emotionally and mentally. It leads to an obsessive preoccupation with food that blinds you to the many other pleasures of life. Dieting makes you feel guilty and depressed about your body and your lack of will power. You can get irritable, angry, and finally rebel against your diet. You start to eat all the food you've been craving until you gain back all the lost weight and maybe some extra. Then remorse and guilt make you hate yourself. You hate yourself so much that you talk yourself into another diet. And the nightmare continues.

## Dieting Doesn't Work

As harmful as dieting is, it might be worth the pain and suffering if it worked once and for all. But it doesn't.

If you're caught in the chronic dieting nightmare like Janice is, you know this is true from experience. You hear about a new diet and get fired up to try it. Maybe you join Weight Watchers™ or Nutri-Systems™ or some other group that's active in your area. While your motivation is high, you stick to it and the pounds start to come off.

You feel good. You're in control of your weight and your life. People say you look great. You wonder why this was such a problem for you in the past. It's easy.

After a few weeks the pounds stop coming off so easily. You're tired of the diet and it isn't working as well. Suddenly the forbidden hors d'oeurves and ice cream and lasagna start looking awfully good. You fall off your diet, either with a crash or with a subtle slide. Sometimes you feel panic as you realize that you're losing control. Sometimes you watch yourself in horror as you eat like a machine that can never be satisfied. Any casual mention of food, even a picture in a magazine, can trigger a familiar sinking sensation of depression and hopelessness.

Maybe you pull up your socks and get back on the straight and narrow for a while. Maybe you don't. Either way, you're eventually off the diet. The pounds creep back on. You end up weighing the same as you did before the diet—or a bit more. You look in the mirror and hate your body.

Even though that diet didn't work, you always have the hope that the next diet will be the one that *does* work. Some day you hope to find the right formula for lifetime weight control. Then all your suffering with your weight problem will be repaid with interest and you'll be welcomed permanently into the ranks of those happiest of happy folk—the slim people.

I hate to dash those hopes, but they are an illusion. You'll never achieve lifetime weight control through dieting. Even established, organized, scientific weight loss programs admit to a 90 to 98 percent failure rate over the long term. The overwhelming majority of their graduates *do not keep the weight off.*

"But," you say, "maybe I'll be in the lucky two to ten percent that *does* keep the weight off." Unfortunately, even that small group is not so lucky. Most of them keep the weight off by continued dieting and constant deprivation. Many slide over the line from chronic dieting into anorexia or bulimia. They do not magically become slim beings who can now eat spontaneously and not gain weight.

It's painful, but you have to face it: the ranks of traditional dieters who can achieve satisfying, lifetime weight control are vanishingly small. To understand why, you need to delve a little further into exactly *why* dieting doesn't work.

## Why Dieting Doesn't Work

If you're like me, you have probably suspected for some time that dieting just doesn't work very well, at least in your particular case. But it's hard to understand why. Common sense tells you that the way to lose weight is to eat less. After all, everyone knows that weight is maintained by how much you eat, right? Eat more and you'll gain weight, eat less and you'll lose weight. It's often reduced to a simple formula, one you've undoubtedly seen before: 3,500 calories equals one pound. To lose a pound, cut 3,500 calories out of your maintenance diet. It's simple and obvious, right?

Well, it's actually not that simple.

### Basal Metabolism Rate

To understand how your body maintains, gains, and loses weight, you need to consider how your basal metabolism rate fluctuates.

Basal metabolism rate is how fast your body uses food in a resting state. "Basal" means the base, the lowest activity level—when you're sleeping or just sitting doing nothing. "Metabolism" means turning food into energy, changing what you eat into movement and body heat. "Rate" just means how fast. The rate can be expressed in calories per minute or hour or day.

In practical terms, basal metabolism rate comes down to how many M&Ms your body burns up to maintain your present weight and keep you warm and breathing while you're slumped in the EasyBoy watching Jeopardy. Let's say that's currently two M&Ms per minute.

If you cut down your intake of M&Ms, your basal metabolism rate will slow down. Your body will become more efficient and it may take only one M&M per minute to keep you alive at the same weight. It's like having a car that gets more miles to the gallon when you put less gas in the tank.

This is one reason diets don't work well. Underfeeding your body gradually slows your basal metabolism rate so that your body actually needs less food to maintain the same weight. During the first week of a diet, the 3,500-calorie-per-pound formula may hold true, and you'll lose a pound for every 3,500-calorie reduction you make in your food intake. But soon your basal metabolism slows down and that 3,500 calorie reduction now results in only three quarters of a pound lost. The longer you stay on a reduced calorie diet, the less weight you lose per week. To put it another way, you will have to eat less and less to lose the same number of pounds each week.

Basal metabolism rate is also responsible for the rapid weight gain you experience after going off a diet. When you go back to your previous food intake, your basal metabolism takes a while to speed up again. You resume eating two M&Ms per minute, but your basal metabolism is still operating at the fuel-efficient one-M&M-per-minute rate. For a while, until your metabolism speeds up, the extra energy from that extra M&M is stored as fat—you gain weight on the amount of food that previously maintained your weight.

This is bad enough, but it gets worse. When you deprive your body by dieting, it tries to restore the missing food by making you very hungry. You crave those M&Ms so much that when you go off the diet, you may eat three per minute for a while instead of your old rate of two per minute. There's even more extra energy available to store as fat.

### Fat Cells and Muscle Cells

The picture gets even darker when you look at what happens to fat and muscle when you diet. When you lose weight on a diet, your fat cells and muscles both shrink. You don't actually decrease the number of cells, just their size.

When you gain weight, you gain almost all fat and no muscle. And your fat cells not only swell up again, but they also start multiplying. You end up with more fat cells than you started with.

So repeated weight loss and gain results in shrinking muscle mass and more fat cells. It's not a simple cycle in which you keep coming around to the same point. It's an upward spiral that keeps getting worse and worse. Every time you lose weight and gain it back, you add new fat cells that you'll never be able to lose. The statement "I can always lose it again" is never entirely true.

### Setpoint

If you think about how your basal metabolism rate changes according to how much food is available, you can see that your body behaves as if it wants to stay within a specific range of weight. This weight range is called the setpoint range.

Setpoint can be defined as your physiologically optimum weight range—what you would weigh if you gave up all dieting and ate spontaneously. This can be a wide range. You tend to stay at the low end of your setpoint range if you eat a balanced, nutritious diet and lead an active life. You tend to stay at the high end of your setpoint range if you eat junk food and get very little exercise.

Your setpoint range is largely inherited. There's nothing you can do to change it. Some of us were meant to be slim, some of us were meant to be plump, and most of us were meant to be somewhere in the middle.

(I use the words "slim" and "plump" here in a purely descriptive manner, without any judgment or criticism implied. In our culture, calling someone fat or plump or stout is usually taken as an insult, whereas it's considered a compliment to call someone thin or slim. In writing this book I discovered that

*there is no neutral word for fat* in the English language
at this time. So as you read further, you'll just have
to remember that when I use words like "fat" and
"plump," no criticism is implied.)

The inherited nature of your setpoint range is bad
news if you want to be slim and your genes want you
to be fat. Fighting to stay below your inherited setpoint range will make your life miserable. When you
fail to maintain your "ideal weight," you'll blame
yourself for being a glutton, for lacking will power,
for being a slob, and so on. And over time you
actually won't eat any more than your slim friends
eat.

This bears repeating. It's a very slippery fact, but
a true one: stout people don't eat any more than slim
people. In 1982, J. S. Garow published *Energy Balance
and Obesity in Man*, in which he reviewed thirteen
studies of the relationship between weight and food
intake. In twelve of these studies, scientists found
that fat people eat the same or less than skinny
people. In only one study did they find that fat people
ate slightly more than slim people. These unexpected
results have prompted duplicate studies to test the
findings, and the results so far have come out the
same:  fat people don't really eat any more than thin
people.

Lifetime weight control begins with accepting this
comforting fact: that you can't change the setpoint
range you've inherited from your parents. No matter
how you fool around with your food intake, your
body will keep coming back to the weight it "wants
to weigh."

There's no way to change your setpoint range. The
most you can do is change your lifestyle so that you

stay at the low end of your natural range. Improving your diet—less fat and sugar, more whole grains and unprocessed foods—will take you about half way. This doesn't mean eating less, just eating better. Significantly increasing your activity level will take you the rest of the way—to the bottom of your setpoint range. That's why this book devotes full chapters to nutrition and increasing activity.

There is a way to *exceed* your setpoint range: chronic dieting and the fluctuations of weight gain and loss that go with it. When you lose weight on a diet, your deprived body makes you hungry and your metabolism gets very efficient in its use of energy. You tend to gain back more weight than you lost. Several cycles of dieting, weight loss, and weight gain can result in you weighing much more than your natural setpoint maximum. Chronic dieting pumps up your weight like a car jack raising a bumper: two clicks up, one click down, two clicks up, one click down, and so on. The only way to flip the switch and let yourself back down to your natural setpoint range is to stop dieting and learn to eat spontaneously again.

Kelly Brownell, a psychologist at the University of Pennsylvania School of Medicine, studied "yo-yo dieters" who went through repeated cycles of weight loss and gain. In 1988 she reported two disturbing findings. First, the dieters she tracked lost weight much more slowly on their second diet than on their first diet. Second, they gained back the weight much more quickly after the second diet than after the first diet. Dr Brownell's theory is that repeated dieting slows your metabolism and makes your body very efficient at storing and conserving fat. Your metabolism tends to stay slow because after repeated dieting you end up with less muscle tissue and more fat tissue, which is less metabolically active than muscle. It remains to be seen whether this metabolic slowdown is permanent or just very persistent.

How much can you lose and still be in your setpoint range? The number depends on several factors: your height, age, frame size, where you are in your setpoint range now, the kinds of food you eat, how much exercise you get, and whether people in your family tend to have wide or narrow setpoint ranges.

For example, Suzanne weighed 190 pounds after years of chronic dieting. She was thirty years old, had a medium frame, and was five feet eight inches tall. She ate junk food and got very little exercise. In other words, Suzanne was probably over the top of her natural setpoint range and had lots of room for improvement. When she stopped dieting and started eating all she wanted of a nutritious diet, she dropped to 175 pounds. Feeling lighter and more vigorous, she started going for walks, dancing, and taking the stairs instead of the elevator at work. She finally stabilized at 160 pounds. That's a range of 30 pounds.

On the other hand, Gini started at 140 pounds when she gave up dieting. She was shorter and lighter of frame than Suzanne. Her diet was just as deficient, but she was accustomed to more daily activity. Improved nutrition and more exercise helped Gini stabilize at 125 pounds—a range of 15 pounds.

Kim gave up dieting when she was very slim. A year of rigid willpower and almost daily workouts at a gym had kept her at 120 pounds, but the cost was too great: she felt cold and hungry all the time, missed periods, had a constant fear of losing control, and experienced wildly fluctuating moods. She began eating more spontaneously and cut back on her fanatic exercise program a little. Kim indulged her cravings and rapidly gained 20 pounds. Then later she dropped a little to a stable weight of 135 pounds. She feels a lot better now.

The point is not how much you can lose. The point is how you can be healthy, happy, and free of obsessions about your weight.

### How To Determine Your Setpoint Range

It's not necessary to figure out your setpoint range to achieve lifetime weight control. You can just stop dieting, eat more nutritious foods, and stay active. The weight at which you eventually stabilize will be, by definition, within your setpoint range. But it's human nature to want to look into the future and know in advance what's likely to happen.

There's no way to tell whether you're within your setpoint range by just looking. It varies from person to person and there are no external indications. Your best clues will come from your medical records. Obtain as much information as you can from all the doctors you have gone to. Make a chronological chart of your age, height, weight, level of activity, and any special diets you were on:

| Age | Height | Weight | Level of activity | Dieting? |
|-----|--------|--------|-------------------|----------|
|     |        |        |                   |          |
|     |        |        |                   |          |
|     |        |        |                   |          |
|     |        |        |                   |          |

Look at the chart and find a time when you had reached your full adult height and had not been on a diet for a long time (ideally, a year or more). The highest weight you reached during this period is probably well within your setpoint range.

Any weight that, as an adult, you were able to maintain effortlessly, without dieting, is probably within your setpoint range. If your records and recollections are complete enough, you'll probably see that you moved slowly up and down in your setpoint range according to the quality of your diet and your level of activity.

However, if you have been fretting about your weight and dieting since adolescence, it will be hard to find a clear pattern. You may never have had a dieting-free year as an adult. Your weight has probably fluctuated wildly above or below your setpoint range. If this is your case, look for a weight to which you always return after a diet. This weight is probably a little higher than the top of your setpoint range. In other words, if you had never dieted you would probably have stayed at a lower weight than the weight to which you always return.

If you are a "successful" dieter who maintains a very low weight for long periods of time by constant starvation, your setpoint range probably begins a few pounds above the weight you are trying to maintain. Hopefully this news will be liberating rather than depressing. It means that you have been fighting your body's natural state, starving and torturing yourself needlessly. You don't have to do that anymore. By giving up your diets and eating spontaneously, you will gain the additional weight that your body needs to be healthy and operate at its optimum performance level. You'll trade your dangerous slimness for healthy self-acceptance and peace of mind.

If you've read all the above and are still confused about your setpoint, look at your parents and siblings, especially any who just eat what they want and don't diet. If your immediate family are mostly slim, your setpoint range is probably on the low side. If your family members are generally stout, then your setpoint range is probably higher than average.

## Who *Should* diet

Not everyone should just stop dieting. Dieting is justified as an extreme measure if obesity is threatening your life. For example, if you are very obese and you also have diabetes or heart disease, a weight loss diet could save your life.

How fat is "very obese?" The chart below offers some estimates. But don't base any serious decisons about dieting on a simple chart alone. If you are very concerned about your weight and other health problems, see a doctor to help you decide.

If you weigh more than the "obesity level" for your sex and height *and you have diabetes or heart disease*, you should seriously consider losing weight by means of a nutritionally balanced, reduced calorie diet, under a doctor's supervision. Once you have dieted down to a more average weight for your height and any immediate health problems have stabilized, you can stop dieting and follow the program recommended in this book.

## Serious Obesity Levels
## Persons Twenty Years and Older

| HEIGHT (Without shoes) | WEIGHT (Without clothes) |
|---|---|
| **Women** | |
| 5′ 0″ | 170 |
| 5′ 1″ | 175 |
| 5′ 2″ | 180 |
| 5′ 3″ | 185 |
| 5′ 4″ | 190 |
| 5′ 5″ | 195 |
| 5′ 6″ | 201 |
| 5′ 7″ | 207 |
| 5′ 8″ | 213 |
| 5′ 9″ | 219 |
| 5′ 10″ | 225 |
| 5′ 11″ | 231 |
| 6′ 0″ | 237 |
| **Men** | |
| 5′ 3″ | 203 |
| 5′ 4″ | 209 |
| 5′ 5″ | 215 |
| 5′ 6″ | 222 |
| 5′ 7″ | 229 |
| 5′ 8″ | 235 |
| 5′ 9″ | 243 |
| 5′ 10″ | 250 |
| 5′ 11″ | 257 |
| 6′ 0″ | 264 |
| 6′ 1″ | 271 |
| 6′ 2″ | 279 |
| 6′ 3″ | 287 |

Fortunately, your chances of losing weight and keeping it off are good if you are very obese when you start. Studies have shown that when very obese people lose weight, they lose more weight, more quickly, and are much more likely to keep it off than people who were just a little overweight to start with.

If you need support in your dieting, consider joining a group or established program. But don't hesitate to try losing weight on your own. Studies have shown that people who lose weight on their own are more successful than those who become involved in a supervised program.

If you *don't* have diabetes or heart disease, don't go on a diet, no matter how heavy you are. Even if you have some other condition that has been traditionally associated with obesity—cancer, hypertension, breathing problems, high cholesterol, arthritis, kidney disease—you shouldn't diet. The danger to your health is probably not immediate enough to justify dieting. Research such as Kelly Brownell's is beginning to show that the stress of fluctuating weight caused by repeated dieting is probably worse for you than the stress of just staying heavy. You'll be better off if you follow the long-term weight control measures in this book and *very gradually* settle into your setpoint weight range.

## In Summary

This chapter has covered a lot of important but complicated material. Briefly, here are the high points:

- Chronic dieting is a harmful, widespread eating disorder.
- Just staying heavy is healthier than repeatedly losing and gaining weight.
- Chronic dieting makes you *fatter* in the long run because of the way your basal metabolism ad-

justs during and after periods of food deprivation.
- Chronic dieting makes you *weaker* in the long
run because with each diet you lose both muscle
and fat, but gain back only fat.
- Stout people don't eat any more than slim
people.
- Your *setpoint* is the weight range, largely inherited from your parents, that is normal and
healthy for your particular body.
- Good nutrition and exercise will keep you at the
low end of your setpoint range.
- Chronic dieting can pump your weight up until
it's above the top of your natural setpoint range.
- The only people who should diet are those who
are seriously obese and suffer from diabetes or
heart disease. If you think you might be in this
category, see your doctor.

# C

# But I'm Too Scared

Have you ever been a victim of binge eating? You can't seem to get enough ice cream, fudge, potato chips, or whatever. You can't get full. Even if you do feel full, you can't stop eating.

It doesn't matter what you tell yourself: "I'm out of control, I'll get fat as a house, how can I do this to myself, I'm no good." In the face of intense cravings, these self-statements make you feel bad but don't make you stop eating.

Or maybe during the binge you aren't conscious of any thought at all—just mindless eating. The self-recriminations come later, when it's too late.

When you consider abandoning all your diets and eating spontaneously, you may fear that your life will beome one long binge. You may fear that you'll blow up like a hot air balloon or become some kind of circus freak. Reassurances to the contrary are little help. The fear is real and keeps you stuck in the dieting rut.

Many fears surround dieting, food, and spontaneous eating. Different people find different things frightening. What scares me might not scare you. What worries you might not bother me. In this chapter you'll have a chance to carefully examine your own, personal fears about weight control. Some of your fears will probably be eliminated by the end of the chapter. Others will probably remain for you to overcome later.

Overcoming your fears about spontaneous eating is worth the effort because getting free of dieting offers great hope as well: hope for a future with no food obsessions, no failed diets, no binging, and no self-hatred; hope for a future of stable weight, self-esteem, and a wholesome enjoyment of food.

By the end of this chapter, you will be able to weigh your fears accurately against your hopes. You'll be able to judge whether spontaneous eating is for you at this point in your life, and you will be able to proceed with confidence if you are ready.

## Common Fears Checklist

Read through this list carefully and check the fears you share. In the spaces provided, write out any additional worries you have that aren't already on the list. Take your time and do a thorough job, because this information is crucial to the decision-making process you'll practice later in this chapter.

### If I Eat Spontaneously

- ☐ **I'll Gain Weight.**
- ☐ I'll look ugly.
- ☐ I'll look old.
- ☐ My health will deteriorate.

☐ My nice clothes won't fit.
☐ I'll have to shop in the big and tall store.
☐ I'll go broke buying all new clothes.
☐ _____

☐ **I'll lose control.**
☐ I'll eat everything in sight.
☐ I'll go crazy.
☐ I'll have a panic attack.
☐ I'll have a heart attack and die.
☐ I'll be terribly depressed.
☐ I'll be a failure in my own eyes.
☐ _____

☐ **I'll be giving up, admitting defeat.**
☐ I'll hate myself.
☐ I'll lose my self-respect.
☐ All my struggles with weight will have been a waste.
☐ I'll have to finally give up the image of a thin me.
☐ I'll be just like my fat parents, sister, brother, or friend.
☐ _____

☐ **I'll be a failure in the eyes of others.**
☐ I'll lose the respect of my family and friends.
☐ So and so will be so mad at me.
☐ My boyfriend or husband will leave me.
☐ My girlfriend or wife will leave me.
☐ My weight-conscious friends will ostracize me.
☐ Strangers will think, "What a fat slob, what a glutton."

- ☐ I'll be setting a bad example for my spouse and kids.
- ☐ I'll lose my job.
- ☐ _____

- ☐ **I'll lose my sexual attractiveness.**
- ☐ No one will want to be with me.
- ☐ I'll be all alone.
- ☐ I won't be feminine anymore.
- ☐ I won't be a real man anymore.
- ☐ _____

- ☐ **I'll have to give up my dieting lifestyle.**
- ☐ I'll have to quit my diet group.
- ☐ I'll have to quit the exercise class.
- ☐ I'll have nothing to talk about with my weight-conscious friends.
- ☐ I won't get to try that new diet I've been hearing about.
- ☐ Without my diet pills, I'll have no energy.
- ☐ I'll have nothing to do without dieting and obsessing about food.
- ☐ _____

- ☐ **It won't work**
- ☐ I can't do it.
- ☐ I'll fail at this like I failed at dieting.
- ☐ Then I'll really be in trouble.
- ☐ The rest of my life will fall apart too.
- ☐ _____

- ☐ **I'm afraid it _will_ work.**
- ☐ I'll feel like a fool for all those years of dieting.

☐ I'll be so angry at all those who encouraged me to diet.
☐ I'll be too happy—I don't deserve to eat freely.
☐ I'll be too attractive—people will make unwanted advances.
☐

_____

☐ **I don't even want to think about it.**
☐

_____

# Common Hopes

Look over your responses to the checklist and see where your greatest fears lie.

People differ, but they're similar too. This section briefly shares some of the hopes—the positive ways of thinking—that others have used to counter their fears about spontaneous eating. Read it carefully and see which hopes you share or might make part of your own strategy for handling fear.

## Gaining Weight

Yes, if you've been starving yourself "successfully" for some time, you will gain weight when you eat spontaneously. Even if you are within your setpoint range when you start eating spontaneously, you might still gain some weight. And there's no denying that the setpoint weight at which you stabilize might be heavier than the "ideal" weight that you have been yearning for all your adult life.

**The real choice.** When you're struggling with the decision to give up dieting for good, don't be fooled into thinking that you're making a choice between being thin and being fat. If you're a chronic dieter at war with your own body, this is not really the choice that confronts you. Being thin is not really an option—at least not the effortless, happy, glamorous kind of thinness you desire. The only kind of thinness you can achieve is the miserable, constantly starving life of the chronic dieter.

So your real choice is not between thin and fat, but between misery and contentment. If you choose "thin," you are really choosing misery—committing yourself to a constant struggle to be thin, with many failures, fluctuating weight, damaged self-esteem, and poor health. If you choose "fat," you are really choosing contentment—allowing your body to stabilize in its natural weight range so that you can be comfortable, well fed, healthy, happy, proud, and finally at peace.

Ironically, most people who give up dieting end up weighing less than the weight that they used to return to after going off a diet. They make the "fat" choice, and end up getting thinner anyway. It's like a Zen paradox—you get only what you give up wanting.

As for the other fears associated with gaining weight—concerns about appearance, health, and having to buy new clothes—they are all largely illusions. Following the steps in this book regarding exercise and nutrition will result in better health and appearance in the long run than you could ever hope to maintain as a chronic dieter. You may end up a few pounds heavier than your previous "ideal weight," but you'll look better, feel better, and be healthier.

When your weight stabilizes within your setpoint range, you can enjoy the luxury of wearing clothes that really fit you well today and will fit tomorrow and next year as well. In terms of your wardrobe, lifetime weight control is a very sensible economic decision. No longer will you have to keep three wardrobes on hand—too big, OK-for-now, and too small. Lifetime weight control is also size control.

*Losing Control*

Dieting can be a satisfying way of taking control of your life, especially if you have low self-esteem. Taking rigid control of what you eat allows you to feel like you're in in control of your whole life. It's a wonderful feeling, during the first week of a new diet, to be able to say "I'm on this terrific new diet, and I've lost five pounds in six days." You're proud of yourself, others are proud of you, and you feel on top of things.

Unfortunately, it's not so wonderful in the fourth or fifth week of the diet, when your enthusiasm and willpower have eroded and the dramatic rate of weight loss has slowed to a standstill. Then you're likely to go off the diet with a crash, suddenly binging on some favorite food.

When you go off a diet that you had great hopes for, it feels like you have lost all control of your life. You feel crazy, self-destructive, and helpless to do anything about it. This can trigger genuine panic, with pounding heart, shortness of breath, dizziness, and so on. Panic symptoms can become so strong that you feel like you're having a heart attack and are in danger of death. This naturally makes you even more frightened and you become trapped in a vicious spiral of escalating fear.

Even if you stick to a diet, lose all the weight you want to, and go back to eating normally without binging, you can gradually become depressed as you notice yourself eventually regaining the weight you lost.

If you've had these powerful feelings of losing control before, then the prospect of no more diets and spontaneous eating can be very frightening. It may seem like you are being asked to give up all control of your life and plunge into a terrifying void.

To conquer this very real fear, you need to do two things. First, do some serious thinking about the nature of control in your life, with the goal of broadening your concept of how you might stay in control. Second, start lifetime weight control very slowly, with emphasis on the word "control."

When you think about control, try to see the long term. Look beyond the latest diet and how you'll look next summer. Instead, consider how you want to feel and look five years from now. Imagine how much better you'll feel about yourself if you can stabilize at a healthy, effortlessly maintained weight. Begin seeing that the way to *really* be in control of your life and your weight is to give up dieting and make slow, positive, long-term changes in your nutrition and activity level. This will do much more for your self-esteem than losing ten pounds on the latest diet and then gaining it all back again. It's another Zen paradox: you have to let go of one kind of false control in order to seize true control.

When your attitude begins to shift and you become ready to try lifetime weight control, start slowly. Follow the directions in the next chapter for easing into spontaneous eating. Go at your own pace so that you can feel like you are retaining control. When fears of binging and losing control come up, remind yourself that you now have permission to eat whatever you want, whenever you want. Remind yourself that dieting and self-denial caused your intense cravings and binging in the first place. As you go longer and longer without dieting, your metabolism will calm down, your cravings will weaken, and your sense of real control over your life will grow stronger.

Going slowly like this, it will take you longer to accomplish the first step and achieve truly spontaneous eating. But it's better to go slowly than to never start.

### Failing Yourself

For years you have been creating and editing an image of yourself as a person who is thin or one day will be thin, a person who doesn't or shouldn't eat certain foods, a person who is fundamentally very different from fat parents or sisters and brothers. When you go to bed at night, you judge yourself according to what you ate or didn't eat during the day: "I was good today" or "I was bad today." You love yourself to the extent that you follow your dietary rules and hate yourself when you break them.

Just opening this book is a big threat to your self-image. Eating spontaneously without a thought about calories is like betraying state secrets to the enemy or abandoning your religious beliefs. It can shake you to the core. It can make you feel that you've given up the battle or become a failure.

The way out of these feelings is to realize that your old self-image was an illusion. The vision of an effortlessly thin you was always a mirage, a dream you fashioned for yourself to help you through the pain of dieting. Giving up that kind of image is a good thing. It frees you to create a new, healthier image based on the true facts about weight and the body you were born with.

Perhaps being heavy bothers you because you don't want to be like other members of your family who are heavy. Being thin or trying to be thin sets you apart from them. In this case, you need to make a list of all the ways in which you are different from them that have nothing to do with weight: your relationships with others, your accomplishments, your taste in clothes or furnishings, your hobbies and interests, your beliefs about love and life—qualities besides mere shape.

### Failing Others

Mothers, fathers, siblings, lovers, spouses, children, friends—they all have their own opinions about you. They may have been hassling you for years about your weight. Their hassling may take the form of constant nagging, heartfelt love and concern, or a walking-on-eggshells silence around the subject of weight.

However expressed, the way others feel about your "weight problem" is a powerful force in your life. Others can determine whether you try a diet or go off a diet, whether you order ice cream or just coffee for dessert, whether you leave this book out on the kitchen table or hide it in your dresser, even whether this book and your program of lifetime weight control will be successful.

With so much riding on the opinion of others, you have to take your fears about failing them very seriously. There is no single piece of good advice that is going to lay those fears to rest once and for all. Each of your relationships is unique, and you will have to deal with the issue of spontaneous eating differently with different people.

Think of all the people who wouldn't like it or wouldn't understand if you gave up dieting and started eating spontaneously. Write down a list of their names.

Some of the names on your list will be people whose opinions aren't particularly important to you. Cross them out.

Other names may belong to people who are very reasonable and will understand once you carefully explain what you're doing. Write "explain" next to their names and plan to talk with them seriously the next time you get a chance.

You may decide that some people just can't be convinced. If you can just avoid them, do so. Put parentheses around their names and plan to stay out of their way.

For those who can't be convinced or avoided, just plan on not telling them anything. They'll probably never notice any changes in your eating behavior. Put square brackets around their names.

And so on. As you cross people off your list or plan how you might handle their reactions, you will probably discover two things. First, the list of important people who really might "lose respect" for you is relatively short. You might even notice that some of your fear is ungrounded—on close examination, many of the people whose respect you value don't really care what you eat or what you wear. You might even have been "projecting" your values on to others, assuming that they were as concerned about your weight as you are.

Second, you are probably left with one or two really important people whose opinions of you really count. These are the ones whose support you will need as you embark on your program of lifetime weight control. In the chapter on meeting emotional needs you'll learn how to get support from these really important people in your life. You can't do it all alone, and you don't have to do it all alone.

### Sexual Attractiveness

Happy, healthy, active people have better sex lives, regardless of their weight, than unhappy, unhealthy people who are constantly dieting and obsessing about their weight. If you can convince yourself that lifetime weight control will make you one of those happy, healthy people, then your fears about losing sexual attractiveness will evaporate.

Worries about heaviness being a turn-off are usually more in your mind than in the mind of a potential lover. The fact is that compatible personality traits, common interests, and mutual caring are much stronger attractions than mere shape. These are the bonds that hold relationships together and foster a good sex life.

But perhaps you have a lover who is also obsessed with weight. Perhaps your lover prefers you unnaturally slim no matter how unhappy it makes you to get and stay that way. If this is so, then your fears about losing sexual attractiveness are justified—and you have some difficult choices to make. If you're with someone who is stuck in the singles bar/*Penthouse* magazine mindset, it will be very difficult for you to eat spontaneously and risk gaining weight and losing the relationship. You will probably have to ease very slowly into your program of lifetime weight control, and your program probably won't be successful until your relationship changes.

*No More Dieting Lifestyle*

Dieting together is fun. Eating together is one of the great human bonding experiences. It brings family and friends together, whether you're splitting a low-cal diet plate or feasting on apple pie and just *talking* about the next diet.

If you've been dieting off and on for years, you probably have lots of friends and acquaintances who are also into dieting. You may belong to a weight loss group or an exercise program that stresses weight loss. Thinking and talking about food is enjoyable. It fills your empty moments. You're never at a loss for a topic of conversation. TV, radio, newspapers, and magazines reinforce your preoccupation with food and dieting. Dieting is a big part of your lifestyle, a component of many habitual attitudes and behaviors that you enjoy, or at least persist in.

If the thought of losing your comfortable dieting lifestyle fills you with fear and grief, you should postpone taking the first step. Wait until you have lined up an alternative social support network and figured out how to keep some of the good things about the dieting lifestyle.

A good way to get support and preserve the social aspect of dieting is to interest someone else in lifetime weight control. Give a copy of this book to your best dieting pals and convince them to try it out with you. Then you can work on spontaneous eating together. If you liked sharing the diet plate with your friends, you'll love eating what you really want together.

If you value the social life centered around a dieting plan or exercise class, find another group to join. Look for a self-esteem support group or an exercise program that will further your program of lifetime weight control, without emphasis on weight loss and reaching an "ideal weight."

Unfortunately, I doubt that any "Lifetime Weight Control" groups will open for business in your local mini-mall as a result of this book. There are no special foods or menus to sell to group members, so there's not much chance for big profits. And this book counsels a slow, long-term approach that doesn't lend itself to special promotions like "Lose Twenty Pounds in Six Weeks for Only $99."

If you take diet pills, your dependence on a dieting lifestyle may have a chemical basis. Giving up dieting means giving up the stimulant effect of appetite suppressants. This can be quite a loss if you have come to count on the extra boost of energy you get from diet pills. Of course, some of the side effects are easy to give up: the jitters, the insomnia, the paranoid anxiety, and the sudden black depression when you finally "crash." You will definitely have to give up diet medications, because there is no way lifetime weight control will work with stimulants distorting your appetite and energy level.

### Pessimism

A history of failed diets can make you very pessimistic. The doubting, self-critical voice in your head says, "This won't work. Even if others could make it work, I never will. I'll fail at this just like I failed at dieting. And then I'll really be in trouble, with nowhere else to turn."

If you find yourself plagued with this kind of thinking, it will help to go back and read the previous chapter again, especially the sections on why diets don't work. Read slowly and try to understand every nuance.

A careful reading will help you realize that you have been swimming against the current. Trying to control your weight by dieting is like trying to survive the rapids of a powerful river by swimming upstream. You can't do it. All your energy is expended in fighting the current, and you stay in the same dangerous place.

Lifetime weight control is like swimming downstream. It's the way the river and your body wants you to go. Going with the flow gets you quickly into quiet waters and safety.

If you follow the directions in this book, lifetime weight control will work. It will work because for once you will be working with your body instead of against it.

However, pessimism may keep you from following the directions. If you find that your doubts are keeping you stuck, forget about weight control for a while. It's the wrong problem to tackle right now. Concentrate on building self-esteem and a positive outlook. Read other self-help books, take a class, get into therapy—do whatever it takes to curb your negative self-talk and see the world in a brighter light.

### Fear of Success

You may actually be afraid that lifetime weight control *will* work. If it works, then all your years of dieting will be in vain. You might feel pretty foolish about wasted time and money and anguish. Or you might be very angry at your mother, father, or partner for years of hounding you about your weight and the necessity to keep dieting.

On a deeper level, success with weight control might bring up complex issues involving self-esteem or sexuality. Not wanting to deal with those issues could keep you from pursuing weight control wholeheartedly. For instance, if you have low self-esteem you might believe, deep down, that you don't deserve happiness and can't allow yourself to succeed. Or if you are nervous about sex, you may feel threatened by the idea of looking healthier and more attractive to members of the opposite sex.

Again, these are real fears and not to be taken lightly. Until you resolve them, you shouldn't rush into the first step of lifetime weight control.

The first step to rooting out fear of success is to acknowledge it. Finding out that you are really a little bit afraid of succeeding at weight control is a powerful insight. It throws light into previously dim corners of your personality. Getting fear of success out into the open weakens it, since much of this fear's power comes from the way it operates behind the scenes, almost unconsciously.

Admitting your reservations about success also focuses your attention away from your weight for the moment. It makes you consider more profound changes that you can work on first: cutting your losses and letting go of the past, clearing up resentment of others who have an interest in your weight, gaining more self-acceptance, and establishing a comfortable sexual identity.

If you fear success, take special care in doing the hopes and fears exercise that follows. Make sure you give full weight to your hopes and don't exaggerate the strength of your fears.

## Hopes and Fears Exercise

It's hard to give up your dream of someday being slender, supple, and sexy. No matter how unlikely, the dream beckons. It seems that as long as you keep dieting, there's always the chance that someday you'll discover the secret of happiness and finally free yourself from fat. If you stop dieting and pursue the kind of lifetime weight control proposed in this book, it means giving up some very pleasant, powerful fantasies.

After reading the previous chapter you have an idea of your probable setpoint range, and it may be higher than you'd like. If so, the urge to retreat back into dreamland can become very strong. You need to resist that urge right now and objectively weigh the arguments for and against dieting, for and against spontaneous eating.

On the next page, write down all the hopes you have concerning dieting—the advantages, benefits, and positive aspects. In the next section, write down all the fears you have concerning dieting—the disadvantages, negative consequences, and pain you suffer when dieting. Next, do the same for spontaneous eating, listing first the hopes and then the fears.

Of course, some hopes and fears are more compelling than others. So, when you have finished listing all your hopes and fears, rank them according to their importance. Then you can add up the scores to see whether your hopes outweigh your fears or vice versa.

# Hopes and Fears Chart

**Importance**
Relatively unimportant = 1
Moderately important = 2
Very important = 3

**Hopes for Dieting**   (Advantages, positive rewards)

_____   _____

_____   _____

_____   _____

_____   _____

_____   _____

_____   _____

_____   _____

_____   _____

_____   _____

_____   _____

total dieting hopes  +  _____

**Fears for Dieting**   (Disadvantages, painful consequences)

_____   _____

_____   _____

_____   _____

_____   _____

_____   _____

_____   _____

_____   _____

_____   _____

_____   _____

_____   _____

total dieting fears  +  _____

**Hopes for Spontaneous Eating** (Advantages, positive rewards)

_____     _____

_____     _____

_____     _____

_____     _____

_____     _____

_____     _____

_____     _____

_____     _____

total spontaneous eating hopes  +     _____

**Fears for Spontaneous Eating**
(Disadvantages, painful consequences)

_____     _____

_____     _____

_____     _____

_____     _____

_____     _____

_____     _____

_____     _____

_____     _____

total spontaneous eating fears  +     _____

Add up your scores for dieting fears, dieting
hopes, spontaneous eating fears, and spontaneous
eating hopes. Compare your own values to see how
you, as a unique individual, view the advantages of
dieting versus spontaneous eating. Remember that

there is no ideal score or preferred ration of hopes to fears.

### Example

Teri was a 28-year-old chronic dieter whose weight had fluctuated from 135 to 175 pounds since she was eighteen. Here is how she filled out her hopes and fears chart.

| Hopes for Dieting | Relative Importance (1-3) |
|---|---|
| Feel like I'm in control | 3 |
| It might last some day | 1 |
| Look good when I'm skinny | 3 |
| Proud when I lose | 3 |
| Others compliment me when I'm successful at losing | 2 |
| Black dress fits | 1 |
| Total | 13 |

| Fears for Dieting | |
|---|---|
| Hungry all the time | 3 |
| Weird cravings | 1 |
| Depressed | 3 |
| Grouchy | 1 |
| Hard to buy clothes—need three different wardrobes | 2 |
| Binges scare me | 3 |
| Afraid of losing control at any time | 3 |
| Hate my body when I'm fat | 2 |
| Catch more colds and flu when I'm skinny | 1 |
| Weight fluctuations hard on my body | 1 |
| Think about food too much | 2 |
| Have to make two dinners—one for family, one for me | 2 |
| Turned off to sex sometimes | 2 |
| Total | 26 |

| Hopes for Spontaneous Eating | |
|---|---|
| Can forget about food, concentrate on life | 3 |
| Improve nutrition | 2 |
| Better resistance to colds and flu | 1 |
| Save wear and tear on my body | 2 |
| Eat what I really want | 3 |
| Fewer cravings and binges | 3 |
| Only cook one dinner | 2 |

| Whole family's nutrition can improve | 2 |
| Really be in control for a change | 3 |
| Improve self-esteem | 2 |
| More cheerful, less grouchy and depressed | 1 |
| Easier to shop for clothes—just one wardrobe | 1 |
| Total | 25 |

**Fears for Spontaneous Eating**

| Hard to give up hope of being a slender person | 3 |
| Fear I'll just blow up like a balloon | 3 |
| My husband will never desire me again | 2 |
| Friends will criticize me | 1 |
| Have to give away my "very fat" and "very slim" clothes | 1 |
| What will I talk and think about if not food and diets? | 2 |
| Total | 12 |

Teri worked hard on her list to get down all the hopes and fears she could think of. When she added up her scores, she saw clearly that the disadvantages of dieting for her outweighed the advantages by a score of 26 to 13. And her high hopes for spontaneous eating surprised her somewhat—25 points as opposed to only 12 points for her fears about spontaneous eating.

The results were even more dramatic when she added together her scores for dieting fears and spontaneous eating hopes: a whopping 51 in favor of trying lifetime weight control, compared to only 25 total points for the sum of her dieting hopes and spontaneous eating fears.

However, Teri wasn't completely convinced by the numbers. "It's easy to be objective," she explained, "when you're sitting quietly with your self-help book, writing things down. But the real world is full of temptations and people who don't understand what you're trying to do."

Dieting was a way of life for Teri and many of her friends. Not having a new diet to talk about and being open to criticism for "giving up the fight" were serious considerations. Also very frightening was the prediction that she might gain weight uncontrollably if she allowed herself to eat spontaneously. Linked to that possibility was the fear that her husband wouldn't find her attractive.

"I can't just write these things down, put a 'three' after them, and forget them." she said. "They're constantly on my mind."

Teri talked over these considerations with her best friend and her husband. She didn't decide to give up dieting until she assured herself that she had their support. And the only way she could talk herself into trying spontaneous eating was to tell herself it was only an experiment. She told herself that she would give it six months and see what happened (not the best attitude for success, since stabilizing within your setpoint range can take much longer.)

But that's the best Teri could do, and fortunately it worked. After six months of eating all she wanted of a balanced diet, she had gone from 165 pounds up to 172, then back down to 167. Her fears of huge weight gains were unwarranted. "But best of all,' she said, "I'm not so obsessed about my weight. Sometimes a whole day goes by and I don't even think about weight. I still intend to learn to cook more nutritious things and get more exercise, but I'm delighted already with how I feel compared to the way I used to be."

## I'm Still Too Scared

If your fears about spontaneous eating still outweigh your hopes for lifetime weight control at this point, read on but don't *do* anything.

Don't make any changes in your life until you have fully absorbed the next chapter, and perhaps have read this chapter all over again. You might want to put the book aside and just think about for a few weeks, then come back to it.

When you feel ready, consider making a small change to your dieting lifestyle, as described in the section of the next chapter on starting slowly with small steps. If you're not ready to give up dieting entirely, perhaps you can just go on a different *kind* of diet next time. If you can't bear to throw out clothes that don't fit, perhaps you can buy just one pretty item that *does* fit and wear it around the house.

One secret to changing your life is to start small and do what you can, even if it's only thinking about change for now.

# 1

# Eat Spontaneously

This is the first step toward lifetime weight control. It's a very simple step, with easily understood instructions: eat whatever you want, as much as you want, whenever you want. Don't diet or restrict your eating habits in any way.

Spontaneous eating may be simple, but it's not easy if you're a chronic dieter. Eating without restraint goes against the rules of every diet you ever heard of. It conjures up images of gluttony, of runaway weight gain, of being laughed at and despised by others—all the fears covered in the previous chapter.

Spontaneous eating will work best if you use the all-at-once method. This means getting rid of all your diet books, diet foods, clothes that don't fit, and so on. It means going off all diets or nutritional regimens designed to control weight. It means eating only what you really want, regardless of how "bad" the food is or how much you've already eaten. Since the all-at-once method is surest and fastest, I've put it first in this chapter.

If the all-at-once method is too frightening, you should try the gradual method described later in this chapter. The gradual method allows you to ease into lifetime weight control a little more slowly. You can wean yourself away from dieting gradually and experience spontaneous eating at first in carefully controlled circumstances. It will take you a little longer to achieve a stable weight, but you'll still be successful.

## All-At-Once Method

In this method, you systematically dismantle your former dieting lifestyle and for a while give up all attempts to control what you eat. There are three steps: cleaning up your environment, stopping all dieting behavior, and eating spontaneously.

### Clean Up Your Environment

This step is very important. By ridding your surroundings of any trace of dieting, you'll get rid of cues that trigger obsessive thoughts about food and weight. You'll make it much easier to stop all dieting behavior and change your point of view to that of a non-dieter. Follow the steps in order and complete each step before going on the the next one so that you don't miss anything.

**1. Measuring devices.** Put your scale on the top shelf of the closet or out of sight in the back bedroom. Make it very difficult to weigh yourself. Use your scale only for weighing growing kids, pets, prize pumpkins, backpacks, and luggage for exotic vacations in small private aircraft.

Put your measuring tape back in the sewing basket where it belongs. If you have a food scale in the kitchen for measuring out diet portions, put it way in the back of a low, awkward cabinet. If you have a little pocket calculator that you use for adding up calories, take it out of your purse and hide it away in a drawer until tax time.

**2. Foods and drugs.** Flush all diet pills down the toilet. Throw the little bottles and any prescriptions away so that you won't be tempted to refill them. Throw out all the diet food that you don't really like to eat for its own sake: fake cookies, protein liquids, nutri-bars, Rye-Crisp, artificial sweeteners, diet sodas, and so on. Keep only food you enjoy eating.

**3. Books and magazines.** Throw away your little calorie counter booklet and all those Weight Watchers® brochures and daily menu cards. Give away all your old diet books and low-cal cookbooks, unless they contain recipes that you really enjoy cooking, serving, and eating. Get rid of all those back issues of magazines that contain diets you thought you might try some day.

*Stop All Dieting Behavior*

This step parallels each part of the previous step. Once your surroundings are clear of dieting reminders, it will be easier to give up old dieting behaviors.

**1. Don't weigh or measure yourself.** Weighing yourself several times a day, once a day, or even once a week is too often. It will only fuel your obsession with weight. The same holds true for measuring your waist, hips, thighs, bust, and so on. Don't do it. Weighing yourself once a month is often enough to keep track of how you are doing in your program of lifetime weight control. Remember, you're interested in the long term now. Daily or weekly weight fluctuations are irrelevant.

Your goal is not only to achieve weight stability, but also to become *disinterested* in what you weigh. How you feel will be much more important, and you may eventually go for several months without weighing yourself.

When you get the urge to weigh or measure yourself, close your eyes and look inward instead. Ask yourself, "How do I feel? Am I comfortable in my body? Do my clothes fit? Am I warm, cold, tired, energetic, nervous? Am I at peace with myself and others?" Your interior experience of well being is your new scale, your new tape measure.

Likewise, don't weigh or measure what you eat. Don't count calories. Don't even try to take smaller portions. Just load up your plate and eat as much as you want. Trying to second guess yourself with "portion control" is just another way to stay obsessed with food and weight.

**2. Don't consume diet drugs or diet foods.** You can never achieve weight stabilization as long as your appetite is distorted by diet pills. Get rid of them and stay off them.

From now on, your sole criteria for eating something will be the fact that you're hungry and you want it, not the fact that it's low in calories. If you *like* cottage cheese and grapefruit for lunch, keep eating them. But if you've been choking down some vanilla-flavored glop or crunching glumly through celery and rye crackers, switch to the spaghetti or sandwich that you really want. Lay off the diet sodas and drink real sodas or fruit juice instead.

**3. Don't read about dieting.** You may have to cancel some magazine subscriptions to achieve this. Magazines and newspapers bombard you with the latest information on who lost how much on which diet. In the grocery checkout line, it's hard to resist peeking into the *Enquirer* to find out how some starlet lost 25 pounds to save her marriage and her part in next season's soap opera.

When tempted to pick up the latest diet best seller, remind yourself, "I'm not interested in diets anymore. I don't diet. I pity those poor, miserable people who are still dieting."

**4. Don't talk about dieting.** When a friend tells you that he or she is on a diet, don't automatically say, "Well good for you. What kind of diet? How much have you lost?" This kind of response feeds the diet obsession—yours and your friend's. Instead, try to have the courage of your convictions. Tell your friend, "Oh, you poor thing. That's too bad. I'll bet you're just starving." Pity, not praise, is the proper response to the news that someone else is dieting.

When someone starts talking about dieting, change the subject as soon as possible. If dieters persist in talking about their diets, tell them, "I'm trying a new approach where I'm supposed to eat spontaneously and not even talk about dieting. Let's change the subject." At the very least, this will focus the discussion on lifetime weight control instead of dieting. Then you'll have a chance to relate some of the facts about lifetime weight control.

*Eat Spontaneously*

It may take you a couple of years to fully accomplish this step, especially if chronic dieting has made you paranoid about food and guilty about the natural pleasure of eating.

Your first goal should be to enjoy eating again. Give yourself permission to eat anything you want, without guilt. Your only criteria for what you eat should be the fact that you want it. Try to eat spontaneously, like you did as a very young child, before you'd even heard of dieting.

Your second goal will be to end preoccupation with food, and your third goal will be to end the battle between your mind and body so that your weight can settle into your setpoint range. The way to achieve these goals is to concentrate on the primary goal: pleasure in food.

Really enjoy what you eat. If you want "bad foods" like cake and ice cream, go ahead and eat them. Don't try to substitute "good" foods for the "bad" foods you crave. Don't even allow yourself to categorize food as "good" or "bad." If you catch yourself doing this, say to yourself, "All food is good. I love my body and I love food."

Later on you can explore more nutritious alternatives to the sweet, rich foods you love. Right now you should concentrate on falling back in love with the foods you have been denying yourself or feeling guilty about eating.

During the first days and weeks of spontaneous eating, you may start calling yourself names like "pig" or "glutton" or "bad." When this happens, remember that you have permission to eat whatever you want, in any quantity. At this point in your program of lifetime weight control, it's your job to eat spontaneously. You're doing what you're supposed to be doing.

When you start blaming yourself for eating too much or eating the wrong things, remind yourself that you are only on step one. You will be working on eating different kinds and amounts of food later, in the nutrition chapter. At this stage, eating a lot of junk food or eating only one kind of food is just fine. Your job at this point is to enjoy food, period. Constantly strive to suspend judgment and concentrate on enjoying food.

When you eat, strive for a feeling of fullness that is comfortable. Eat enough so that you feel satisfied, but not so much that you feel stuffed. But don't worry if you make some mistakes and starve or stuff yourself sometimes. When it comes to knowing when you're satisfied, you are probably out of practice.

Watch out for a tendency to ask yourself, "Am I *really* hungry?" Hunger is mediated by certain areas of the brain and blood sugar levels. When you feel hungry, it's impossible at the moment to tell whether the feeling of hunger is "real" (based on physiology) or "imaginary" (based on some emotional need). When you first attempt to eat spontaneously, assume that all hunger is real hunger. Remember that your first goal is to enjoy food, not to psychoanalyze yourself. You'll deal with the "why?" of your hunger in a later chapter.

At first, you will probably become even more obsessed and crazy about food. You will be afraid of running wild in the caloric jungle and blowing up like a balloon. It's normal to have these thoughts. Tell yourself, "Now I'm going crazy about food, right on schedule." Remind yourself that the frightening thoughts will soon pass, while the benefits of the efforts you are making will be with you the rest of your life. You're working for long-term results now, and your scary thoughts are a short-term reaction that you can get past.

If you've been dieting for a long time, you'll probably experience strong cravings for all sorts of previously forbidden foods. Go ahead and indulge the cravings. They will fade as you progress in your lifetime weight control program.

**Weight gain.** If you've been dieting continuously to maintain a weight below your setpoint range, then you'll gain weight when you start eating spontaneously. You might also gain weight if you have been dieting off and on and you are within or above your setpoint range. Your weight will be reflecting the over-stimulated appetite caused by chronic dieting and the metabolic changes caused by fluctuating weight.

If you do gain weight, or if you just feel worried about it, come back to this book. Read the previous chapter on handling fears and read the next chapter on self-acceptance.

Tell yourself that any appreciable weight gain is probably temporary. You will end up weighing what is healthy and right for your body. Remind yourself that you are looking to the long term now.

When you think about the likelihood of gaining weight, try to resist the falsely reassuring thought "I can always diet it off again." If you allow yourself to entertain the notion of possible future diets, you'll never be free of your weight obsession. When you have this thought—and you undoubtedly will have it often at first—counter with a self-statement such as "I am through with diets. I love my body in its natural, healthy state."

**Relapses.** Don't worry if you backslide and go on a diet again. Forgive yourself, stop dieting, and start reading this book again, especially the last chapter on sticking to it. You may have to chip away at your weight obsession over a number of years. You may need to go more slowly than the pace you originally set for yourself. Consider some of the gradual methods covered in the next section.

## Gradual Method

If the thought of abandoning dieting entirely and eating spontaneously is too frightening, you can use the gradual method. This involves the same basic steps covered above, but you ease into them slowly, building confidence as you go.

*Improve Your Environment*

If you are a chronic dieter, you have probably surrounded yourself with many items that serve to remind you of your weight and dieting. If you can't bring yourself to make a clean sweep at this time, at least make a start by discarding or hiding away a few of these dieting reminders.

Instead of putting your scale or your measuring tape away in a dark closet, just move it. Put it behind a door or in a room that you don't visit very often. When the urge to weigh yourself arises, you'll have to make a little more effort to get to the scale.

If you use a pocket calculator to add up calories, leave it at home sometimes and make yourself use a pencil and some paper. You may have a lot of extra calorie charts, diet books, or magazines with interesting diets that you mean to look at some day. If you can't make yourself give them away or throw them away now, at least put them into a drawer or cabinet where you won't see them often.

If you use diet pills, try to take fewer. If you use special low- cal foods like diet sodas, protein drinks, or low-sugar baked goods, replace one of these items with a small amount of something more nutritious that you really like.

### Improve Your Dieting Behavior

You may feel that you're not ready to give up on dieting yet. Perhaps you want to diet to "get down to" some predetermined weight before you start following the directions in this book. You may even agree intellectually that diets don't work and it's probably best to try the all-at-once method of spontaneous eating, but just don't feel emotionally ready—the thought is too scary or you just don't feel convinced at the "gut level."

That's fine. Even if you're dieting now or plan to diet again, you can prepare for lifetime weight control by limiting the damage that a diet is likely to do. You can choose a type of diet that will be gentler on your body and less likely to set you up for rapid weight gain.

**1. No drugs.** Prescription diet pills are powerful stimulants that speed up your metabolism and suppress your appetite. Over-the- counter brands are a little safer only because they are a little weaker. Diuretics and laxatives provide an illusionary weight loss by eliminating fluids that your body needs to stay healthy. Prolonged use of these drugs is just not good for your body or your emotional equilibrium. And when you stop taking them, your appetite and weight come right back. If you do nothing else to improve your dieting behavior, at least stop taking such drugs.

**2. No "crash," starvation, or single-food diets.** If you must try another diet, at least stay away from drastic regimens where you only eat 600 calories a day or only eat oat bran and celery. Also avoid fasting entirely for two or three days to "shrink your stomach" or "clean out your system" before starting on a diet proper. All these strategies put a tremendous strain on your system. You suffer intense hunger, strong cravings, and various physical symptoms like weakness, dizziness, and cramps. Your suffering is pointless because when you go off the diet, as you must eventually, your lost weight almost always returns.

**3. Consider a slow, traditional weight loss diet.** This is the kind of diet where you eat a reasonable number of calories from a restricted but nutritionally balanced list of foods. Weight comes off more slowly and the cravings aren't so bad. This kind of diet is still not good for your body, but at least the damage is slight and the weight rebound later on will be smaller.

**4. Better: Make a permanent diet change** This is where you say, "No more ice cream" or "Always a salad instead of starch at dinner" or "Only one pat of butter per meal." This approach still lets you eat until you're satisfied, and it tends to improve your nutrition so that you feel better as well as lose a few pounds. You can keep this up for a long time and abandoning such rules usually doesn't mean you'll gain back any more weight than you lost.

**5. Even better: Practice programmed eating.** This means that you follow a rigid menu for each meal, with no substitutions. The meals are balanced nutritionally, with low fat and low sugar. You can make up your own or join a support group that gives you the menu. Many groups these days even sell you the food, ready to pop into the microwave oven and serve. This approach can be expensive if you join a group and buy special food, but you do get a lot of support. Try to find a plan that lets you eat until you're satisfied. When you go off such a plan, you'll still probably gain back some weight, but more slowly than if you had been on a more extreme diet.

**6. Best: Replace dieting with exercise and consciousness raising.** Maybe you're ready to give up dieting, but you feel you have to do *something*. In that case, take an exercise class or join some kind of support group that will let you share your concerns about weight without encouraging you to go on another diet. The exercise will increase muscle and decrease fat, making you leaner and perhaps a bit lighter. It will do this in the safest, gentlest way possible, and you'll feel much better physically. Talking to others will support your growing readiness to give up dieting for good, eat spontaneously, and pursue the other steps toward lifetime weight control.

### Controlled Spontaneous Eating

It's a bit of a paradox, but you can ease into spontaneous eating by controlling when you do it, where you do it, with whom you do it, and so on. Obviously, spontaneous eating is not going to work really well until it's truly spontaneous, in all areas of your life. But you can benefit from trying it out in limited, reassuring circumstances first.

To start with, choose one place and one time to try spontaneous eating. You might plan to go to a new restaurant, some place where you have no history of conflicts about food. Or you might want to try spontaneous eating first in a favorite little cafe that you associate with good times and where you feel relaxed. You can plan to take a trusted friend or family member, or go by yourself if you'd rather not have anyone watch what you eat. If you have someone with you, you can share your plan with him or her or not, depending on whether enlisting support or keeping quiet feels better to you.

Before your trial meal, don't think too much about what you'll order or what it will feel like. Tell yourself, "Just this once, I can have exactly what I want, and I won't know what that is until I get there."

When you arrive, take a deep, relaxing breath and open the menu. Let your eyes roam over the selections until you find something that appeals to you. Undoubtedly, you'll have thoughts like "Oh no, I can't have cream sauce—too fattening." When this happens, take another deep breath and tell yourself, "Stop that! I can have it if I want it." You might close your eyes for a moment and imagine the sight and taste and smell of a dish and see if it seems like you'd enjoy it.

Don't forget to consider salad, soup, appetizers, dessert, and so on. You don't have to have them to prove anything to yourself, but you don't have to deprive yourself either. Just this once, price and quantity is no object. You should order what you really want. If you want to taste several items, go ahead and order them.

Avoid making apologetic comments to your companion or the waiter "I shouldn't have this, but ... I'll be sorry ... It's so fattening ..." and so on. It's best not to say anything about your selection. Just order with a straight face.

When your food comes, eat what you want of each dish. If you want more, order it. If you have too much to finish, you can take the leftovers home in a doggy bag or just leave them on the plate for the waiter to take away. Above all, don't undermine your experience by talking about the calories, thinking about eating too much, or planning how you'll starve yourself tomorrow to make up for eating so much today. Concentrate on the flavors, textures, and aromas. If you have a companion, say whether you like or don't like the food, but don't converse about weight or diets.

Congratulate yourself when the meal is over, even if you slipped a few times and felt bad about eating what you really wanted. If this was a positive experience, plan to return to the same restaurant to do it again. Or plan to try the same technique at a different restaurant.

If your first trial was a disappointment, ask yourself what you can do to improve your odds of success. Perhaps you should try a different cafe, or take someone with you next time, or go alone, or change the setting to dinner at a friend's house. Experiment until you find a place, a time, or a social situation in which you're comfortable eating spontaneously.

Once you're comfortable in one situation, expand your horizon by repeating the experience more often or in different places.

Rob's example is a good one. He was a radio-therapy technician who first tried spontaneous eating at lunch in the hospital cafeteria. In the past, he always took the same thing—a muffin, a banana, and a cup of tea—to avoid temptation. One day he just drifted along the steam tables, picking what he wanted. He ended up with some Chinese stir-fried vegetables, a piece of fried chicken, some tapioca pudding, and a cup of tea. This was more than he usually had, but it was delicious and he really enjoyed it. Later he started blaming himself for "eating like a pig," but he managed to remind himself that it was just a trial, and a successful one at that.

A couple of days later, Rob repeated the experience. He chose pork roast, french fries, two helpings of jello salad, and a cup of tea. He was surprised that he didn't finish the second jello. "As a charter member of the clean plate club," he told me later, "I was very surprised. I realized that if I could have anything I wanted, I could also choose *not* to eat something I didn't really want to finish."

The next time Rob tried spontaneous eating, he was at a potluck party on the weekend. He allowed himself to sample everything that looked good and went back for seconds on the chicken wings and the cheesecake. He explained:

> When I ate whatever I wanted, I was always a little nervous that I would run amok and eat everything in sight. I thought I'd do that to make up for all those dry muffins and underripe bananas. But when it actually came down to it, knowing that I could eat it all somehow made it possible to pick and choose. I ate more than I would if I had been being "good" and sticking to my usual rules. But I ate less than when I suddenly decide to hell with the rules and really

pig out. I didn't feel as out of control as I thought
I would.

Soon Rob was allowing himself to choose foods
spontaneously for breakfast and lunch. He still re-
tained his rules about dinner and snacking in front
of the TV at night. Then after about three months, he
gradually gave up on his dieting rules and started
eating spontaneously all the time.

Six weeks before his vacation in Mexico, Rob suc-
cumbed to temptation and went on a 1,100-calorie-a-
day diet:

> I just had to fit into my old red trunks and be
> able to walk down the beach without sucking it
> in so much. And it worked, sort of: I lost twelve
> pounds before I left, gained six back in the two
> weeks I was in Mexico, and gained another
> seven after I got back. Now I'm through with
> diets. It's time to get back into jogging, learn to
> accept my body more, and eat more vegetables.

*In Summary*

To ease into spontaneous eating, you need to
remove some of the dieting reminders from your
surroundings, choose healthier diets when you must
diet, and gradually experience spontaneous eating
more and more often.

Learning to eat more spontaneously will undoubtedly bring your old fears to the surface many times.
You'll worry about gaining weight, losing control,
losing attractiveness, experiencing the disapproval
of others, and so on. At those times, you should
return to this book and the exercises you have done.
Remind yourself of the nightmare of dieting and of

your commitment not to suffer like that again. Review your analysis of your hopes and fears surrounding dieting versus lifetime weight control.

As you work your way through the rest of this book, you'll gain insights and skills that can finally put your fears at rest. If you get discouraged or "backslide" along the way, don't give up hope. Setbacks are normal and expected when you're trying to make a major change in your life. Keep your eye on the long term and remember that progress is made in a series of leaps, plateaus, and valleys—not in a straight line.

# 2

# Accept Yourself

Imagine that you're a little child, four or five years old, snuggling in your mother's lap. (If your real mother was absent or not the snuggling type, imagine an ideal mother figure.) Feel her arms around you, the warmth of her legs and stomach under you, the softness of her breast where you lay your head. You feel safe, secure, loved. Everything is right with the world. You are perfectly OK, just as you are.

Did you ever watch the kid's show "MisterRogers' Neighborhood"? Many adults are initially put off by Fred Rogers' style. But kids love him because he tells them what they most want to hear: "You always make each day special for me, just by being you. You're the only one like you in the whole world, and people can like you just the way you are."

You never outgrow your need to hear this message: that you are unique, that you are fine just as you are, and that people can like you just the way you are. This is the essence of self-acceptance. When you accept yourself you value yourself without conditions. You say, "I'm OK, period," instead of "I'd be OK if I could just lose forty pounds."

Does this mean that you should just accept being fat and give up any attempt to control your weight? Absolutely not. Self-acceptance doesn't preclude self-improvement. When you say "I'm OK," you're saying that you like and value yourself as a human being, with all of a human being's strengths and weaknesses.

Self-acceptance actually makes self-improvement easier. When you accept yourself as a fallible human being, it's easier to look at your good and bad points. It's easier to tell yourself the truth. You can examine things like your eating habits, your food preferences, your sedentary lifestyle, and your appearance with greater objectivity. You can face the facts without beating yourself up, making excuses, or denying your weight problem.

Regardless of how much you weigh or how bad your eating habits are, you can accept yourself. This chapter will guide you by exposing some of the cultural obstacles to self-acceptance, presenting some reassuring facts about weight, and providing step-by-step exercises. The most important part is the exercise section. Commit yourself right now to actually *doing* each exercise, not just thinking about it or "running through it" in your mind.

## Cultural Obstacles to Self-Acceptance

Being obsessed with weight is painful in many ways. There are the physical discomforts of hunger while dieting, being stuffed after a food binge, weakness, fatigue, missed periods, cold sensitivity, and cramming yourself into too-tight clothes. You can eventually eliminate this physical pain by stopping all diets, eating more spontaneously, improving nutrition, wearing only clothes that fit, and so on.

Then there are the psychological agonies of weight obsession: depression over being fat, guilt about eating "bad" foods, fear that you'll lose control, and anger at your lack of will power. With persistent effort you can gain self-acceptance, learn to meet psychological needs more effectively, and reduce this kind of pain to a minimum.

But there's one source of pain that you can't avoid or eliminate entirely: the attitudes, assumptions, and expectations of a culture obsessed with weight and appearance.

In America and most other western countries, we glorify slimness and laugh at fatness. Just flip through the TV channels at any time of day or night. The heroes and heroines are slim. The fat people are mostly comic relief. Advertising consistently glorifies slim body types and makes fun of heavy body types.

The fashion industry glorifies outright skinniness. Adolescent models are dressed and made up to look like adults to sell an image of how every woman should look. No matter that the best designs will fit only one quarter of the population. Never mind that adolescent skinniness is inappropriate, unhealthy, and impossible to attain for most women. If you're lucky enough to have the "in" kind of body, you can flaunt the latest style. If you're perfectly normal, you have to go to the "large" store and take what you can get.

Everywhere you look there is evidence of our cultural obsession with appearance. Beauty contests, body builders, and pornography are blatant examples. More subtle indications are the use of beautiful models to sell auto parts or office furniture, shoes and clothes that constrict and hamper free body movement for the sake of style, and politicians who are more concerned with providing photo opportunities than debating the issues.

Our culture has a lot of myths and moral judgments about fat people. Everyone "knows" that fat people are jolly, fat people are neurotic, fat people are gluttons. No matter that studies have repeatedly shown that there is no correlation between weight and personality type, weight and mental health, or weight and significant variations in food intake.

In our society you can discriminate against fat people and get away with it. It's about the only kind of discrimination that is still socially acceptable. For example, you could decide not to rent a house to someone because she's a "disgusting fat slob." Most people would understand and support your decision, whereas they would be shocked if you said you didn't want to rent to a "dumb nigger." The idea behind this double standard seems to be that fat people are somehow to blame for their fatness in a moral way. Few people realize that the tendency towards fatness is inherited to almost the same degree as skin color.

The basic problem with our cultural assumptions is that bodies are seen as ornaments, not instruments. In other words, the first and only judgment of someone's body is an aesthetic one: Is this body pretty, slim, attractive? This ornamental view can lead you to say "I'm too fat," meaning that you're too fat to be considered attractive in our society.

But an instrumental view of bodies asks not how do you look, but what can you *do*? The judgment is practical instead of aesthetic. You may be too fat to be considered conventionally beautiful, but are you too fat to breathe? To move? To walk? To work? To make love? Are you too fat to live your life? Obviously not, because you *are* living your life.

Overcoming the cultural obstacles to self-acceptance means fighting to be seen as a fully functional being instead of a Christmas tree ornament. This can be especially difficult for women. Our male-dominated society *prefers* women to be weak, childish ornaments—not mature, fully functional adults. If you give up dieting and strive instead to be healthy and happy at a higher weight, you may receive heavy criticism for being "unfeminine" or even crazy.

The cultural obstacles to self-acceptance are difficult to overcome because they exist both inside and outside you. Even if you uproot and reform your own personal ideas about acceptable weights and shapes, our culture's crazy and dangerous ideas about weight still surround you, inescapable and unchangeable, constantly challenging your hard-won self-acceptance.

## Some Reassuring Facts

### Metabolisms Differ

You've probably heard the hardnosed, "tough guy" line about losing weight, maybe from a doctor or other scientifically trained person of authority: "Overeating causes overweight, so to lose weight you've got to eat less. At your height and age, you should be eating xxxx calories a day to maintain weight. For each 3,500 calories you cut from that maintenance diet, you'll lose a pound."

This is so simplistic it's useless. Basal metabolism varies from person to person according to sex, age, height, the ratio of muscle to fat, and activity level. And even if all of these factors are equal, there is still a variation of 15 percent on either side of the norm. This means that you can have two women, both 25 years old, five feet six inches tall, with the same ratio of muscle to fat on their bodies, the same weight and figure, and the same level of daily activity. One of them could consistently eat 30 percent more food than the other one, and neither would gain or lose weight. Both would have "normal" basal metabolisms. One might cut back 2,000 calories and lose a pound, while the other would require a 4,000 calorie reduction to lose a pound.

The fact is that some of us are meant to weigh more than others. Your heredity and metabolism dictate a certain weight range that is normal and healthy for you. Imagine that you went out and weighed the first thousand people you encountered who were your sex, age, and height—then plotted their weights on a graph like the one below.

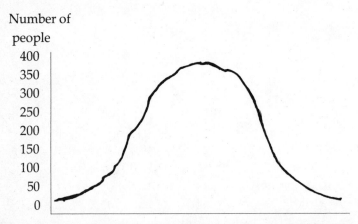

Number of people

The curve that you would undoubtedly plot would be a classic bell curve, since most people would fall in the middle of the weight range and fewer and fewer people would fall at the extreme ends. This is a normal distribution when measuring a single characteristic of a large group—whether it's weights of humans, heights of corn plants, or how far ping pong balls roll when dropped repeatedly from the same height.

The curious thing about weight distribution in our culture is that people don't feel comfortable being in the middle or high sections of the curve. Everybody wants to get into the skinny, low-weight end of the bell curve, a distribution that only widespread famine or some other disastrous event could bring about.

### What About Those Weight Charts?

You see them in most books and magazines about weight loss, health, exercise, or nutrition: those depressing charts that invite you to look up your age and height and read across to your ideal weight or recommended weight range. The result is almost always bad news.

Where do these charts come from? Why do the recommended weights on some of them seem so low? Are they accurate? Are the recommended weight ranges the same as setpoint weight ranges? If you're over the maximum weight, does that mean that you're obese and headed for health problems?

The first such chart was published in 1959 by insurance companies trying to establish acceptable weight ranges for life and health insurance applicants. They sorted several years worth of insurance applications by sex, age, and height, and then averaged the weights reported by the applicants. For the most part, the data used was whatever the applicants reported, not what was confirmed by a doctor's examination.

Well, you know that heavy people are going to shave a few pounds off their actual weight when filling out an insurance application. And thin people don't want to sound too skinny. So the first weight charts had unrealistically, low weights and narrow weight ranges. In 1983, most charts were revised upwards across the board by ten to fifteen pounds. Did everybody suddenly get fatter? No, the insurance companies finally wised up and started looking at more objectively verified weights.

But the newer charts are still nothing more than averages. There is no correlation between the reported weights and the relative *health* of the insurance applicants. The "recommended range" for each sex, age, and height is determined by a formula that arbitrarily decides where to make the cutoff on the low end and the high end—where to slice the bell curve of reported weights. That arbitrary cutoff point has nothing to do with health. It's just a statistical convenience.

Sixty million Americans think they have a weight problem, many of them because they've been brainwashed by these charts for years. But only half of them are right. Real scientists, as opposed to insurance actuaries, are now discarding the charts and doing away with terms like *normal*, *average*, *ideal*, or *recommended* weight. They favor the notion of "natural weight"—the weight at which you are comfortable, the weight that you can maintain effortlessly, without any conscious effort to eat more or less than you feel like eating.

Thinking in terms of natural weight gives you a much wider range of weights that could be healthy for you. A more realistic chart showing possible healthy weights might have weight ranges 20 percent wider than the one devised in 1983. It would look like this:

## Possible Healthy Weights
## For persons twenty years and older

| HEIGHT (without shoes) | WEIGHT (without clothing) |
|---|---|
| **Men** | |
| 5'3" | 106-155 |
| 5'4" | 110-160 |
| 5'5" | 113-164 |
| 5'6" | 117-171 |
| 5'7" | 121-177 |
| 5'8" | 125-183 |
| 5'9" | 128-187 |
| 5'10" | 132-191 |
| 5'11" | 135-196 |
| 6'0" | 139-201 |
| 6'1" | 142-207 |
| 6'2" | 146-211 |
| 6'3" | 149-215 |
| 6'4" | 152-219 |
| **Women** | |
| 5'0" | 90-130 |
| 5'1" | 93-133 |
| 5'2" | 96-137 |
| 5'3" | 99-140 |
| 5'4" | 102-144 |
| 5'5" | 105-147 |
| 5'6" | 108-151 |
| 5'7" | 111-154 |
| 5'8" | 114-158 |
| 5'9" | 117-163 |
| 5'10" | 121-168 |
| 5'11" | 124-173 |
| 6'0" | 127-178 |
| 6'1" | 130-183 |

"But," you say, "those ranges are so broad as to be meaningless." Well, that's just the point. No chart can tell you your natural weight. The only way to determine your natural weight is to stop dieting, eat when you're hungry, and see what happens.

### A History Lesson

Back in 1911, anxious mothers told their daughters: "Eat, eat. You're skin and bones. Nobody wants to marry a scrawny woman." Fat was in. Full figures were the only kind considered beautiful. A typical fashion model from today would have been considered pitifully undernourished.

Society values whatever is hardest to achieve. When life is strenuous and food expensive, then fat is considered the sign of beauty and success. When life is easier and rich food abundant, everyone wants to be slim.

Look at illustrations in old books or ads in facsimiles of old magazines. You'll see that our obsession with slimness is a relatively new fashion. Look at nudes painted or sculpted by artists through the ages. You'll see that the full figure—what we'd probably call fat today—was the norm and the standard of beauty for centuries.

This history lesson reminds you of something that is easy to forget these days: people come in many shapes, and no one kind of body is intrinsically better or more beautiful than another. Adult women's abdomens and bottoms and hips are *supposed* to be rounded. It's just in the last few decades that fashion has arbitrarily said it's no good to look like an adult woman—that everyone should look like an undeveloped teenager.

# Exercises

## Come to Terms With Mirrors

Take off all your clothes and stand in front of a full-ength mirror. Look carefully and objectively at every part of your body. Turn around and use a hand-held mirror to look over your shoulder and see what you look like from the back.

Try for an honest but noncritical assessment of all your different features: the parts you like as well as the parts you don't like. Start at the top of your head and work systematically down to your toes. You will probably find many neutral or positive aspects of your body that you usually ignore in favor of focusing on the bulges. Perhaps you don't like your chin or thighs, but your ears and hands are OK, and your eyes and shoulders are actually attractive.

Don't keep score. Your goal isn't to judge yourself like a horse at a show. The goal is to love yourself, regardless of shape or size. Try to get into a loving, accepting frame of mind. Even if it sounds like a lie, say to your image, "I love you just as you are."

When the usual negative thoughts arise ("What a slob … God, I look like a cow … No one could love me."), remind yourself of the goal of the exercise. Tell yourself, "No negativity … I accept my good and bad points … I can face facts … People can love me just the way I am."

If you tend to avoid mirrors as a general rule, do this exercise daily for a couple of weeks, then weekly after you can view your image calmly and compassionately.

On the other hand, some people tend to check every mirror and shop window to see how they look. They pat up the extra flesh under their chins, smooth their dresses over their hips, fluff up a loose top, turn this way and that to find the slimmest angle, throw out their chests a little, and suck in their tummies.

If you are prone to this kind of mirror obsession, do the mirror exercise just once. Then put away or cover up all your mirrors. Purposely avoid looking at yourself in mirrors. If you catch yourself glancing in car or store windows at your reflection, immediately focus your awareness inside yourself. Instead of assessing your outward appearance, examine your *inner experience* at the moment. Ask yourself, "How do I feel inside, right now?" Healthy? Strong? Excited? Sick? Sad? Anxious? Happy? Tired? Or what? Remind yourself that your body is *your* instrument for living *your* life, not just a decoration on parade for others to look at.

### List Strengths and Weaknesses

This is really a continuation of the mirror exercise, expanded to cover more than merely physical attributes. You'll need a pen or pencil to do this exercise, and some extra sheets of paper if you don't want to write in the book.

**1. List weaknesses.** On the chart that follows, jot down your most worrisome weaknesses in each area of your life:

**Weaknesses ("Bad" Points)**      **Strengths ("Good" Points)**

PHYSICAL

_____      _____
_____      _____
_____      _____

PERSONALITY

_____      _____
_____      _____
_____      _____

INTELLIGENCE

_____      _____
_____      _____
_____      _____

SOCIAL LIFE

_____      _____
_____      _____
_____      _____

WORK/SCHOOL

_____      _____
_____      _____
_____      _____

FAMILY

_____      _____
_____      _____
_____      _____

SEX

_____      _____
_____      _____
_____      _____

OTHER

_____      _____
_____      _____
_____      _____

**2. Edit weaknesses.** Go through your list looking for pejorative, judgmental language. Change these harsh labels into neutral, objective descriptions of your body and your behavior. For example:

| *Change this:* | *To this:* |
|---|---|
| Giant hips, pot belly | 42-inch hips, 38-inch waist |
| Flabby thighs | Cellulite on backs of thighs |
| Grossly overweight | 172 pounds |
| Stringy, greasy hair | Thin, oily hair |
| Wallflower | Slow to approach strangers |
| Spineless jellyfish, no guts | Unassertive, don't stand up to Jack or Mom |
| Slow, clumsy | Needed much practice to learn stick shift and knitting |
| Dumb | C's in math and science |
| Lazy | Sometimes one to two days late with papers and reports |
| Compulsive eater | Sometimes eat when not really hungry |
| Lousy in bed | Comfortable with only one way of making love |

The idea is to change negative labels into objective, accurate descriptions of your body or behavior at specific times, in specific place, and with specific people.

Doing this exercise will help you become more truthful and objective about yourself and hopefully show that you have many strengths and good qualities that you tend to overlook.

**3. List strengths**. Jot down your strong points: the things you do well and the parts of yourself you are proud of (or at least content with).

If you have trouble thinking of strong points, look for inspiration among your weak points. Every minus implies a plus. For instance, "bottom sticks out like a caboose" implies that some other part of the train doesn't stick out. So look for well-formed shoulders, a sensuous back, or shapely ankles. Likewise, "shy with strangers" can make you think of how warm and open you are with a special friend. "Often too tired to make love" may prompt you to admit that when you're not too tired you're sometimes spontaneous and playful in bed.

Find a strong point to correspond to each of the weak points that bother you most. You'll use these weak/strong pairs to compose affirmations in the next exercise.

Here is an example of a strengths versus weaknesses chart completed by Sharon, a 32-year-old divorced waitress and mother of two children in grade school.

First, here's how she edited her first list of weaknesses.

### Weaknesses ("Bad" Points)

| *Change this:* | *To this:* |
|---|---|
| PHYSICAL | |
| - OVERWEIGHT | – 159-163 lbs. |
| - WEAKLING | – Pant going upstairs, lifting suitcases |
| - NEARLY BLIND | – Myopic |
| PERSONALITY | |
| - PUSHY | - Sometimes very outgoing |
| - GULLIBLE | - Trust people on short acquaintance |
| - NOT VERY THRIFTY | - |
| INTELLIGENCE | |
| - UNEDUCATED | - 3 years high school |
| - DENSE | - Takes me a while to learn new things |

- INTIMIDATED BY SMART  -
  PEOPLE

### SOCIAL LIFE

- SILLY WHEN DRINKING   -
- GO OUT WITH BUMS       - Have picked 3 losers
- SPEND TOO MUCH TIME  - Spend 2-3 evenings a week
  IN BARS                               in bars

### WORK/SCHOOL

- ALWAYS LATE                   - Often late
- FLIRT                                 - Talk a lot with customers
- GETTING NOWHERE          -

### FAMILY

- LEAVE KIDS ALONE TOO - Leave kids alone 2-3 even-
  MUCH                                  ings a week
- NEVER CALL DAD             - Seldom call dad
- CAN'T AFFORD TO TAKE  -
  KIDS TO DISNEYWORLD

### SEX

- JOKE A LOT ABOUT IT       -
- TOO EASY                         - Sometimes get intimate
                                            quickly
- TOO FAT TO BE  SEXY       - 159-163 pounds

### OTHER

- HAVEN'T BEEN TO
  CHURCH IN YEARS

Next, Sharon composed a strength to counter each
weak point:

*Weaknesses ("Bad" Points)*      *Strengths ("Good" Points)*

### PHYSICAL

- 159-163 lbs.                          + Dress well
- Pant going upstairs, lifting   + Can work long hours,
  suitcases                               dance all night
- Myopic                                + Pretty Eyes

### PERSONALITY

- Sometimes very outgoing     + Spontaneous
- Trust people on short           + Optimist
  acquaintance
- Not very thrifty                   + Generous

## INTELLIGENCE

| | |
|---|---|
| - 3 years high school | + Interested in current events |
| - Takes me a while to learn new things | + Good with hands, tools |
| - Intimidated by smart people | + Jack's smart and he really likes me |

## SOCIAL LIFE

| | |
|---|---|
| - Silly when drinking | + Rarely really tie one on, don't hurt anyone |
| - Have picked 3 losers | + Dumped them pretty quick |
| - Spend 2-3 evenings a week in bars | + Haven't missed a PTA meeting or parent's night this year |

## WORK/SCHOOL

| | |
|---|---|
| - Often late | + Willing to work overtime |
| - Talk a lot with customers | + Big tips |
| - Getting nowhere | + Big tips again, pretty content |

## FAMILY

| | |
|---|---|
| - Leave kids alone 2-3 evenings a week | + Always food in icebox, neighbors to call |
| - Seldom call dad | + Always a birthday card |
| - Can't afford to take kids to Disneyworld | + Love my family and that's what counts |

## SEX

| | |
|---|---|
| - Joke a lot about it | + Good sense of humor |
| - Sometimes get intimate quickly | + Not recently |
| - 159-163 pounds | + But I still enjoy sex when it happens–generous lover |

## OTHER

| | |
|---|---|
| - Haven't been to church in years | + Believe more in people than in Jesus |

### Compose and Use Affirmations

This exercise will be easy if you have done a thorough job on the previous exercise.

An affirmation is a short, positive statement that you say to yourself to counteract your habitual negative thoughts. It acts like a posthypnotic suggestion, reminding you to be objective, accept yourself, and focus on your positive aspects. Like good hypnotic suggestions, affirmations should be short, with no negative words, and be in the present tense.

To get started, select three or four of your most depressing weaknesses, and write down the corresponding strength in the form of an affirmation. Here are Sharon's first attempts:

> I dress well.
> My eyes are pretty.
> I'm a generous, spontaneous optimist.
> People like being around me.

Notice how Sharon combined three strengths ("spontaneous," "optimist," and "generous") into a powerful affirmation about her personality. And she summarized her social strengths in one simple, clear statement about people liking to be around her.

The best time to use affirmations is when you're starting to get down on yourself with thoughts about your weaknesses and shortcomings. When your "bad" points pop into your mind, you should immediately correct them with objective, edited statements, and then use your prepared affirmations.

For example, Sharon was driving to work in the morning when she caught herself thinking "I'm so overweight, I'm a weakling, I'm broke all the time." She remembered the objective way she had worded her list of weakness and the affirmations she had written down the day before. She gave herself this little pep talk while waiting at a stop light:

> Now wait a minute here. I'm about 160 pounds right now, but I dress well and I have pretty eyes. I may not be a weight lifter, but I can work all day and dance all night when I'm in the mood.

And so what if I'm not a saver? I'm a generous, spontaneous optimist

It's a good idea to make up one or two additional, more general affirmations about your weight, for use when you get a sinking feeling of discouragement or guilt or fear without any obvious negative thoughts. Here are some affirmations that have helped others:

I love myself.
I'm doing my best.
I love my body.
I accept everything about myself.
I trust my body.
My body will settle down in time.
My body moves well.
My body serves me well.
I can let go of anxiety.
I can rise above depression.
I shake off false guilt.
Weight is just weight—not sin.
I just eat when I'm hungry.

When you have a good stock of affirmations—thirty or more—you're ready to start using them systematically in your life. Here are the best ways to use your self-acceptance affirmations:

**Hourly repetition.** This works especially well when you are first learning to use affirmations. Each morning, get two or three blank three-by-five file cards. On one side, write a negative statement that you typically make to yourself. On the other side, write one of your affirmations designed to refute or replace that statement. Do this on two or three cards, using the negative statements that seem to be bothering you most recently. Here are some examples:

I'm too fat./I can love my body just the way it is.

I eat too much junk food./I allow myself to eat
  what and when I want.
Weak, no willpower./I love and take care of
  myself.

Carry these cards with you wherever you go. Once
an hour during the day, take your cards out and read
them. First read the negative statement on a card,
then turn it over and read the positive affirmation.
Read each card in turn, out loud if you are alone.

The next day, fill out a fresh set of cards, even if
you use the same statements. Change the statements
used on one of the cards each day for variety. Feel free
to make changes in the statements according to your
experience with them the previous day.

This exercise requires a certain time commitment
and some inconvenience, but it's great for providing
the repetitive reinforcement needed to make an affirmation part of your automatic way of coping with
negative thoughts.

**Loop tape.** Buy a fifteen- or thirty-second loop
tape, the kind that is used in automatic telephone
answering machines. Record three or four affirmations on it in a slow, calm voice. Keep talking, repeating your affirmations, until the tape is full. Listen to
this tape on your portable tape player or in your car.
The tape will repeat for as long as you want, drum-
ming your positive self-statements into your ear.

Do a tape with all "I" statements: "I am a lovable
person. I have a graceful walk…" Then try recording
the same affirmations as "you" statements: "You are
a lovable person. You have a graceful walk…" This
will add variety, and you may find that you prefer
one way of phrasing your affirmations over the other.

**Writing self-dialogues.** Affirmations are a way of
challenging and changing the negative, critical voice

that you have inside your head. You can accelerate this process by writing out an affirmation and using it to stimulate a dialogue between your negative voice and your healthy, positive side. Here's an example of how it works.

1.

*Affirmation:* I'm generous, outgoing, and optimistic.
*Critical Inner Voice:* Yeah, you'd give away your life savings, if you had any.
*Healthy Response:* So what, what I have is mine to give.

2.

*Affirmation:* I'm generous, outgoing, and optimistic.
*Critical Inner Voice:* You're simple minded, you mean.
*Healthy Response:* No, I choose to see the bright side and that's my right.

3.

*Affirmation:* I'm generous, outgoing, and optimistic.
*Critical Inner Voice:* People take advantage of you. That's stupid.
*Healthy Response:* You're not going to get me down. I like people, plain and simple.

4.

*Affirmation:* I'm generous, outgoing, and optimistic.
etc.

The instructions are simple. Write your affirmation on the first line. On line two, write whatever negative response comes to mind to invalidate your affirmation. Write a healthy, positive comeback on the third line. Then start all over with the same affirmation and see what negative response comes up this time. Respond to it and continue. To get maximum value out of this exercise, persist until you've done twenty or thirty repetitions of your affirmation.

You may find that your negative voice starts to repeat itself. This is good, since it may mean that you are zeroing in on a negative self-statement that you habitually make. Don't worry if your comebacks start to repeat or if you can't think of any reply beyond "Shut up!" or "Leave me alone!" It takes great insight and strength to tell your inner negative voice to shut up, especially after repeated assaults.

**Reminder signs**. This is another form of repetition, designed to bring your affirmations into awareness at odd moments, when you don't expect them. Put up little signs made from three-by-five cards or Post-It® notes. Put "I trust my appetite" on the fridge. Put "Acceptance" on the dresser mirror. Put "My body takes me where I want to go" on the sun visor of your car. Put "I am a mature, adult person with many talents" inside your briefcase. Keep "I can wait out anxiety" in your purse.

You may think it silly or embarassing to post these little signs all over the place. But they really work, silly or not. One way to avoid embarassment is to use more subtle reminders. Get some small kids' stickers or price stickers from a stationery store and put them up instead of signs. Only you will know that the green price sticker on your clipboard means "I know how to take time to relax." Only you will know that the unicorn sticker on the handle of the dustpan is there to remind you that you're a loving mother who does a lot of important little things for her kids.

**Active integration**. This is a combination of the hourly reminder exercise and the writing exercise. It's a powerful way of keeping your affirmations fresh and meaningful.

Each day, select three of your strengths from the exercise earlier in this chapter. Write each one on a

three-by-five card and take the cards with you wherever you go that day. During odd moments throughout the day, look at your cards and think of times in
your past when you exhibited the three strengths. If
you think of a good example of a strength, write it
down on the appropriate card.

Your goal is to have at least two examples of each
strength by the end of the day. Set aside some time in
the evening to complete the exercise if you haven't
written enough examples by then.

Here's an example of active integration.

*Calm in a crisis.* 1. Like the time Christie cut
her head and I took her to the emergency room.
2. When I took over Jean's class on a moment's
notice and did fine.
*Friendly.* 1. I know the butcher, the mailman,
and most of my neighbors by name and enjoy
visiting with them. 2. Three different people in
class asked me to do a team project with them.
*Creative.* 1. My poem was accepted for the
literary quarterly last term. 2. When we went
back east for Christmas, Jim wore the sweater I
designed and knitted.

This exercise transforms your list of strengths
from a mere list of words into specific memories.
These memories help you remember what your
strengths are, believe that you really possess them,
and realize that your strengths really make a difference in the quality of your life.

**Conversational reform.** Monitor your conversation as well as your internal monologs. Instead of
running yourself down, include your affirmations in
your conversation. For example, Sharon would often

meet her friend Brenda for drinks after work, and spout off in this vein:

> Jesus, the bums I've been out with. You'd think I'd learn. I'm just so dense, I don't get it. They tell me night is day and I believe it. So gullible. Of course, beggars can't be choosers. Look at me. Who wants to go out with the fat lady from the circus?

After she had spent some time listening to her loop tape, filling in her file cards, and listing memories of times she showed her strengths, Sharon became very conscious of the negative tone of her gripe sessions with Brenda. She worked hard to make their talks take on a more positive tone:

> Listen, I'm through going out with bums. I'm too trusting sometimes, that's just my nature. But I don't have to settle for the first guy to come along with a good line. I may be heavier than I'd like to weigh, but I'm no bag lady—I know how to dress. I'm setting my sights a little higher these days.

**Recreating affirmations.** As you repeat affirmations, they may lose their original meaning and power. When an affirmation "wears out," make up a new one to take its place.

### Take Care of Yourself

Increase your physical pleasure and decrease your physical discomfort as much as possible. Show that you accept and love yourself by being good to yourself. Treat yourself like the worthy, deserving person you are. Self-care can take many forms. Start with these basics:

**1. Wardrobe reform.** Go through all your clothes and shoes. Get rid of anything that's too small, too big, or not pleasing to you. Give stuff away, sell it, loan it out, hide it in a trunk, or stuff it in the back of the guestroom closet. Just get rid of all the items that you can't wear right now so that you'll stop thinking about them.

Don't wear tight jeans, lifts in your shoes, high heels, girdles, push-up bras, and other nonfunctional items. They'll just fuel your obsession with weight. When you wear constricting clothing, it constantly makes you feel fat, setting off repeated negative thoughts that scuttle your self-esteem.

Consider how the way you dress might be intensifying your obsession with weight and your dissatisfaction with how you look. If you find some connection, try wearing the opposite of what you usually wear. If you usually wear tight clothing and high heels, wear something looser and more confortable. If you hide in baggy clothing, wear something more tailored and revealing, but still comfortable. If you never dress up, try dressing up more. If you always dress to the nines, go for a more casual, comfortable style.

Buy something new that you really like, something that really fits your body right now. Resist the impulse to squeeze into the next smaller size and resist thoughts like "It'll fit fine when I lose five pounds."

**2. Grooming.** Again, break out of an unsatisfying rut by doing the opposite of what you usually do. Move from extremes to a reasonable middle ground. If you spend hours on your hair and makeup and nails, cut way back on the primping. Go with minimal makeup, natural nails, and a simpler hairstyle.

Take a fresh look at your body as something that must do things from the inside out, rather than an ornament that must look a certain way on the surface.

If you habitually skimp on grooming, give it more time and attention. Get a really good haircut and return for another soon. Take leisurely baths or showers and use lots of shampoo and conditioner. Use whatever lotions or cleansers your skin needs. Trim and clean fingernails and toenails carefully. Get a manicure or facial. Take the time to dress carefully in clothes and accessories that match. Shine your shoes, mend rips, and replace missing buttons. Remember, you are a valuable, worthy human being and deserve to look and feel nice.

**3. Health**. If you're a woman who suffers from cramps or premenstrual syndrome, get all the help you can to ease or eliminate your symptoms: doctors, Motrin®, accupressure, visualization, herbs, whatever. Try everything. There's nothing that will alienate you from your body faster than having it turn on you monthly and cause you pain.

Whatever nagging symptom or chronic complaint you have, get it looked at and fixed. Get to work curing and caring for your body. You won't be successful at accepting and loving yourself if you ignore your body's warning signals or postpone treatment.

Get the food, exercise, and rest you need to maintain health. Valuable, worthy, deserving, self-accepting people don't run their bodies into the ground.

**4. Give yourself gifts.** As a worthwhile, totally OK being, you deserve special treats (and I don't mean chocolate decadence). Buy that leather jacket. Take that dream vacation. Go to that special concert.

Pampering or stimulating your body is especially important. Go for a horseback ride, a hot tub, a massage, a hike in the mountains, a walk through the botanical gardens.

Treats don't have to be expensive. Give yourself a gift of fifteen minutes to daydream, a stroll in the park to see if the daffodils are out, one lottery ticket, half an hour's browsing in a book or antique store.

### Resist Brainwashing

This is the hardest exercise because it never ends. Cultural obstacles to self-acceptance are always there.

Don't read magazines that glorify skinniness or push dieting. Be wary of TV shows and ads that imply that fat is bad and slim is good. Don't let the media brainwash you into hating your body because it's the "wrong" shape.

Clean up your own act. Censor your remarks about who's too fat, who ought to drop a few pounds, how much you'd like to lose, and so on.

Expand your aesthetics so that you can begin to see full figures as beautiful. Look at old statues and paintings in a museum or library art book. Imagine how babies must prefer cuddling up to a soft, round person over being clamped in the grasp of a hard, bony person.

Send a donation to or join the National Association to Aid Fat Americans: NAAFA, Box 43, Bellerose, NY 11426. NAAFA is a nonprofit organization that advances the cause of heavy people across a broad front: educational newletters, a weight consciousness workbook, lobbying, fighting discrimination in hiring and health insurance, objecting to offensive ads, support groups for women and singles, a computer dating service, and a mail order book program. The membership fee is only $35.

# 3

# Determine How and Why You Eat

Have you ever had a banana split to celebrate the end of final exams? Have you ever rewarded yourself for finishing a project by going out for a big dinner? Have you ever been disappointed in love and consoled yourself with half a package of cookies? Have you ever made fudge at midnight? Sent out for pizza because you were just too beat to cook or think up something more wholesome? Have you ever been ill at ease at a party and caught yourself gobbling hors d'oeuvres to keep your hands busy and look like you're having a good time?

Do certain foods go with certain places and activities? Beer and ballgames, candy and movies, ice cream and grandma's house?

There are many reasons for eating besides being hungry and needing to sustain life. This chapter will help you uncover where, when, how, and why you eat. It will increase your awareness of the needs that eating fills for you, so that you can start filling non-food needs with something other than ice cream.

Just reading through this chapter will give you some interesting insights, but they will mostly concern your past behavior patterns. To accomplish real change, you need to do the exercises diligently. Doing the exercises develops your minute-by-minute awareness of your needs, so that you can recognize nonfood needs quickly when they come up.

## Daily Eating Diary

This isn't the fancy, leather-bound kind of diary. Get seven three-by-five cards, one for each day of the next week. The cards are simple, cheap, and easy to carry. Their small size doesn't give you enough room to get really obsessive about your food intake. If you find that you can't get a whole day's food on one card, you're being too detailed.

On each card, put four headings across the top:

*When     Where     What     Thoughts and feelings*
                              (both before and after eating)

Each morning, put a fresh card in your purse or pocket. Right after you eat something, whip out your card and jot it down: the time, where you are, what you ate, and what you happened to be thinking about or feeling at the time.

If you forget to write on your card after eating, do it as soon as you remember. Don't go to bed at night without completing your card for the day.

Don't try to alter your usual eating habits so that you'll look good on paper. Of course, the mere process of monitoring your intake will have some effect on your behavior, but try to eat when, where, and what you usually eat.

Don't get obsessed with the monitoring process: avoid noting portion sizes, amounts, or calories, and stop after one week.

Here are three sample cards filled out by Rachel, a forty-year- old pasteup artist.

| When | Where | What | Thoughts and feelings |
|------|-------|------|----------------------|
| 10:00 | Cafe | Coffee cake, tea, fruit | Tired, but good time talking to Jim. |
| 1:30 | Cafe | Turkey sandwich, fries, shake | Beat, read paper, felt guilty about shake after. |
| 6:00 | Home | Crackers and cheese (lots) | Need to relax and have a bite. After–ashamed. |
| 9:00 | Home | Peach cobbler, tea | Tired, after: depressed that I never did get around to making dinner. |

| When | Where | What | Thoughts and feelings |
|------|-------|------|----------------------|
| 7:45 | Home | Three biscuits, apple, banana | Up early, lots of energy, feel good. |
| 12:00 | Home | Bread, stew, milk, cookies | Glad to have house all cleaned up. |
| 6:00 | Home | Apple | Bored, waiting around for Jim to pick me up. |
| 6:30 | Home | Crackers | Ditto. |
| 8:30 | Ballgame | Hotdog, coke, fries, ice cream, peanuts | Dull game, only fun is to eat. After: bloated, feel stupid. |

| When | Where | What | Thoughts and feelings |
|------|-------|------|----------------------|
| 8:15 | Home | Granola, banana, coffee | Looking forward to Anna's wedding. |
| 11:45 | Home | Tea, cookies, licorice | Anxious to get going to the wedding. |
| 1:00 | Wedding | Mushroom caps, champagne, veggies, lox, sandwich, cake | Happy for Anna, good party. |
| 8:00 | Jim's | Pizza, beer | Feeling cozy, but alarmed at how much junk I had to eat today. |

Rachel immediately noticed patterns in her eating.
She tended to eat when she was bored—waiting around for her boyfriend, sitting through a dull ball-

game. Her food choices were worst when she was tired or anxious—cheese and crackers instead of a real dinner after a hard day's work, candy while worried about getting to a wedding on time. She ate most sensibly when she was active and involved in her life. She ate more when she was depressed or anxious. She often felt depressed and anxious *about* her weight, but those emotions didn't seem to change her behavior.

To help you analyze your own food diary, here is a checklist of common poor eating patterns and reasons for eating other than hunger. Mark any that apply to you and fill in your unique patterns in the spaces provided. For most problem eating behaviors, tips are suggested for changing the "food environment" or otherwise altering your habits.

### When

☐ **I eat when it's time.** Breakfast in the morning, lunch at noon, dinner at 6:30. I've always eaten three square meals a day, whether I feel hungry or not. *Tip:* If practical, change the times of your meals around. When you do sit down for a scheduled meal, pause before filling your plate to ask yourself, "How hungry am I? Exactly how much of each food do I want?"

☐ **I eat whenever food is available.** It's a knee-jerk reaction: see food, eat it. It doesn't matter if I've just finished a big dinner and I'm stuffed. If there's dessert, I eat it. If they passed around little trays of dog biscuits, I'd probably eat them too. *Tip:* Make food the signal not to eat, but to look inside yourself and assess your hunger. Then go ahead and eat if you're hungry.

☐ **I eat whenever I haven't eaten lately.** It's been a few hours since I last ate, so I must be hungry, so I eat. I seldom ask myself if I'm really hungry.

☐ **I eat whenever others are eating.** I eat for social reasons, not because I'm hungry. Sometimes I eat to be polite. Somebody has gone to a lot of trouble to prepare food and I feel it's only polite to eat. I don't want to offend my host or hostess. *Tip:* Sharing food with friends and loved ones is a special pleasure that you certainly should not deny yourself. But the pleasure comes as much from the sharing as from the food. You can eat only as much as you really want and still share in the conversation, the good fellowship, the laughter, and so on. Tell yourself, "I don't have to polish my plate to be liked." When pressed to take seconds or thirds, say "No thanks. It's so delicious that I'd love to have more, but I'm just too full."

☐ **I eat when I'm with certain people.** It's become a custom to have pizza with the softball team and to go out for a big brunch with Dave and Marge. *Tip:* Try ordering a salad with your pizza and eating the salad first. Ask your friends for support in your efforts to improve your nutrition. Suggest menu changes. Or do nothing—these little traditions are very satisfying and they probably don't make much difference in the long run.

☐ **I eat when under stress.** When I know it's going to be a tough day, I automatically pull into the donut shop and stock up on the way to work. There's nothing like a sugary, greasy apple fritter to help me face the pile of work in my in-box. *Tip:* It's common to crave carbohydrates—starchy, sugary foods—when under stress. This is because soon after eating carbohydrates, your endocrin system releases serotonin into your bloodstream. Serotonin is a chemical that acts like a tranquilizer, making you sleepy, less sensitive to pain, and calmer in stressful situations. The next chapter will go into some detail about ways to relax and handle stress without reaching for the fritters.

☐ **I eat certain foods when I'm doing certain things.** Beer goes with cigarettes, Hershey bars always go with me on hikes, movies call for popcorn and a Coke, and I can't watch the eleven o'clock news without my hot chocolate. *Tip:* Don't make extravagant promises to yourself about giving up certain foods or certain activities forever. That way leads to the dieting rat race. Instead, when you go to the movies or the ballgame, take only enough money for the tickets and maybe a *small* amount of your favorite food. If you eat a lot while shopping, try going out with only credit cards and no cash for snacks. At the weekly card game, try putting the snacks in another room and taking a break for food. This will disassociate the eating with the card playing, and make you more aware of how much you are eating, whether you're really hungry, and so on. Tell yourself, "I do one thing at a time. I read, then I eat. I eat a snack, then I watch TV."

☐ **I overdo it at holidays.** I'd never make four kinds of potatoes for a regular meal, but at Thanksgiving our family's got to have them boiled, mashed, scalloped, and candied with baby marshmallows. And heaven help you if you don't eat some of each. Then there are all those little chocolate gold coins around at Hanukah. I've always got one in my mouth. *Tip:* If it's only once a year, why worry? On the other hand, maybe the Christmas eating season for you starts right after Thanksgiving and carries through New Year's Day. In that case, you've got a problem. But a successful solution lies not in rigid resolutions as the holidays approach, but in a gradual, year-round change in attitudes, a slow shift toward better food choices as explained in the chapter on nutrition.

☐ **I tend to eat at other times:**

_____

_____

*Where*

☐ **I overeat at home, where nobody can see me.** I eat tons of junky food that I'd be embarrassed to be seen eating at a restaurant. *Tip:* Practice good nutrition at the shopping stage. Go to the store when you're full, not when you're hungry. Don't buy the junky snack foods that you find so irresistible. Don't let others in your family bring them into the house. Again, this is a difficult change in buying and eating habits that will only be accomplished over the long term as you learn more about nutrition and actually come to *prefer* more nutritious foods. Don't expect an overnight conversion to take place.

☐ **I eat in front of the TV.** It's automatic: dump some corn chips in a bowl, pour a drink, flip on the TV. *Tip:* Keep all your food in the kitchen and eat only in the kitchen, the dining room, or some other designated area. No more candy dishes, fruit bowls, or nut cups scattered around the house. Avoid the TV. Remove all comfortable, soft sofas and chairs from the TV room. Banish food from the TV area.

☐ **I eat all the leftovers at home.** I can't stand to see food go to waste. *Tip:* Cook less. Get one of those "cooking for two" cookbooks and learn how to make small amounts of stew, spaghetti, and other favorites that tend to get out of hand. If you do make a lot of something, immediately divide the leftovers into small portions and toss them into the freezer for future meals. After dinner parties, try to send some of the leftovers home with your guests.

☐ **I love to cook.** Fancy dinners at home are the worst. I taste and sample and nibble and snatch little morsels while I'm cooking and then eat a full meal on top of it when it hits the table." *Tip:* Get your spouse or kids to taste things for you. Practice judging seasonings by smell or by smaller and fewer tastes. Get a "light and healthy" kind of cookbook (not a diet cookbook) and try cooking more nutritious dishes. Finally, don't worry about it so much. As you put your lifetime weight control program into action, the nibbling and tasting will take care of itself.

☐ **I overeat in restaurants.** They give such big portions. I want to get my money's worth. I don't want to look stupid by ordering all this expensive food and leaving it on my plate. Besides, if I didn't eat it all, the waiter or waitress might feel offended. *Tip:* The waiter couldn't care less how much you eat. Try splitting meals with someone else—you order an entree and they order soup and salad. Ask for child-size portions, even if you have to pay full price. Ask for a doggy bag and take the excess home for your lunch tomorrow. Or just steel yourself to leave what you don't want on the plate. Stuffing yourself with unwanted food is more of a waste that leaving it on the plate.

☐ **I overeat at parties** The goodies taste so great. Even when it's not so good, eating the food eases the social tensions. It keeps my hands busy and makes me look like I'm having a good time even when I'm actually nervous and sort of lost. *Tips:* Remind your-self that there are other things to do at parties besides eating: dancing, talking, people-watching, snooping around other people's houses, and so on. If you want to keep your hands full and look busy, then empty ashtrays, offer to get drinks for other people, carry empties back to the kitchen, and so on. At your own parties, include healthy foods like raw vegetables. Make substitutions to slow down your eating. For example, you'll eat a lot fewer peanuts if you have to shell them.

☐ **I overeat other places:**

_____

_____

*What*

☐ **I crave sweets.** I can't resist them. I just stuff myself. *Tip:* If you are or have recently been under your setpoint weight, you might be experiencing "extended taste responsiveness." When your appe-tite is in this condition, sweet foods keep on tasting good long after you would normally have your fill. Even in binge quantities, the sweets can't satisfy your craving. The solution to sweet cravings is a long-term one, involving no more dieting, a gradual shift to more nutritious foods, and increased physical activ-ity. Meanwhile, try to keep sweets out of your imme-diate environment to make it harder to indulge your cravings. This advice applies equally to the other cravings listed below for fatty, salty, or spicy foods.

☐ **I crave fatty foods.** The fried chicken and pud-ding seem so rich and soothing.

☐ **I crave salty foods.** I'm a sucker for potato chips, salami, salad dressings, and so on.

☐ **I crave spicy foods.** If it's not Mexican or Thai, forget it.

☐ **I crave other foods:**

_____

_____

### *Why I Eat*

(Note: The "whys" of eating are complex, inter-twined, and fascinating. You won't find a lot of quick-fix tips here. Save your responses to these items for the next chapter, which suggests ways to fill the needs that overeating is filling for you now.)

☐ **I eat for pleasure.** *Tip:* Nothing wrong with that. Face it, eating is one of life's greatest pleasures. Your body is designed to enjoy eating, even after you've had enough to satisfy your immediate hunger, sustain life, and maintain a given weight. Food goes on tasting good for a little while after you're "full." That's nature's way of encouraging you to store up a little extra fat against lean times. The problem arises when your life is so bleak that eating is almost your *only* pleasure. Then you store up more than just a little fat against lean times. Your natural biological mechanism to survive famine becomes the royal road to obesity. The long-term answer is in the next chapter on fulfilling your needs appropriately with something other than food.

☐ **I eat to ease loneliness.** I spend a lot of time by myself, and eating is solace in my solitude.

☐ **I eat to ease depression.** When I'm feeling blue, eating comforts me and picks me up a little.

☐ **I eat to ease anxiety.** Eating takes my mind off my worries and reassures me somehow. As long as I can eat, everything will be OK in the end.

☐ **I eat to relieve boredom.** Eating gives me something pleasant and positive to do. When I'm eating, I don't have to come up with something to fill the time.

☐ **I eat to reward myself.** It's like when I was a kid: when I was good, I got something nice to eat. I still operate that way. Without special foods as a reward, I wouldn't accomplish a lot of things in my life: going to the dentist, doing the taxes, paying the bills, returning phone calls to people I don't like ... the list goes on and on.

☐ **I eat to reexperience my mother's love.** It's corny, but true. When my mom wanted to comfort me or encourage me or show me she cared, she made me one of my favorite things to eat. To this day, whenever I eat ravioli, cherry jello, or rocky road ice cream, I feel like I'm being taken care of by my mom. I feel loved and safe.

☐ **I eat to punish myself.** I'm such a mess, such a failure, that I don't deserve to be slim and happy. I give myself what I deserve: too much food, too much fat, plenty of misery.

☐ **I eat to punish others.** If certain people didn't treat me so bad, I wouldn't have to eat so much to compensate. It's really their fault. It serves them right if I'm fat and unattractive. They get what they deserve. I'll be damned if I'm going to suffer through diets and hunger with no support from those ingrates. Sometimes the very act of eating is a good way to express anger—really biting and chomping down on the food. I may be heavy, but that just means I get to throw my weight around.

☐ **I eat to rebel.** This society has a disgusting, sexist image of women. We're supposed to be slender, delicate sex objects concerned about nothing but making ourselves attractive to men. I refuse to buy into that by changing my eating habits and losing weight.

## Reasons for Staying Overweight

While you're considering when and where and what and why you eat, consider the possibility that you may sometimes overeat because you want to stay overweight. I know this sounds strange, but bear with me for a moment and keep an open mind.

If being heavy is as ugly and awful and totally unthinkable as our society says it is, why are there so many heavy folks? Why don't they all go on starvation diets, get slim, and stay slim? Because being heavy isn't totally bad. There are actually some advantages to being heavy, and some reasons why people stay overweight—even people like yourself who sincerely desire the benefits of lifetime weight control.

Most of the reasons for staying overweight aren't particularly *good* reasons, but they are *real*—real enough to keep you fat or keep you on the weight gain/weight loss pogo stick for years.

People's reasons for staying overweight tend to be unconscious or only partly conscious. The reasons often involve social anxieties or emotional problems that are so threatening that you shy away from even thinking about them. This reluctance keeps the reasons for staying overweight in the background, where they can't be evaluated, can't be exposed as weak reasons, and can't be discarded so that you can proceed with a successful program of weight control.

This next step is a tough one. Carefully, with an open mind, ponder the checklist that follows. See if any of these common reasons for staying overweight are lurking in the back of your own mind. As you check off any pertinent reasons, start to think about the changes of attitude you would have to make and the risks you would have to take if you allowed yourself to let go of these dubious "advantages" of staying overweight.

☐ **I stay overweight because I need to be big.** Being slim means being little, skinny, and weak to me. I secretly, deep down, want to be big, strong, and powerful.

☐ **I stay overweight to give myself space.** Being fat means that I take up a lot of room. I have wide boundaries. I can keep others at bay. I can cushion myself from the world. The real me is safe in here, at the center.

☐ **I stay overweight so that others will pity me.** Being overweight means that people pity me and give me lots of sympathy.

☐ **I stay overweight to explain why no one loves me.** My weight is a good reason for not having a lover. It explains why friends let me down, why people have left me. I can understand why people wouldn't want to get close to someone as fat as me. If I lost weight, I'd lose my excuse. If I lost weight and people still didn't love me, that would mean that I'm basically unlovable. I can't risk finding that out.

☐ **I stay overweight to avoid having to form relationships.** Finding someone to love who would love me in turn is so overwhelming that I can't even contemplate doing it. As long as I'm heavy, I can put it off. I don't have to take the risk of rejection or embarrassment. I don't have to learn to do what I suspect I wouldn't be very good at.

☐ **I stay overweight to keep busy.** When you're overweight, you have lots to do: worrying about your weight, feeling guilty, feeling depressed, complaining, going on diets, going off diets, talking about food and diets, reading about them. Honestly, if I achieved lifetime weight control, what would I do with all the free time?

☐ **I stay overweight to avoid social engagements.** As long as I'm too fat to be seen in public, I can avoid being seen in public. If I lost weight, I'd lose my excuse for not going out.

☐ **I stay overweight to avoid sex.** As long as I'm so heavy, the opposite sex will leave me alone. If I lost weight, I might attract unwanted sexual advances. Others might expect me to pursue them. My current partner might want to do things in bed that I don't want to do. I myself might be tempted to stray outside my current relationship and get in a big mess. It might bring up painful memories of early sexual abuse that I'd rather not think about. The statis quo may be dull and a source of dissatisfaction, but it's safe, familiar, and risk-free.

☐ **I stay overweight to avoid competition.** Lots of people in my age group and class are constantly competing with each other in sports, for sexual partners, in the job market, for promotions, for prestige. Being overweight gives me an excuse for not trying. When I must compete, being fat gives me an explanation for why I lose. If I lost weight, I'd have to compete on my own merits, and that's terrifying.

☐ **I stay overweight to justify my other bad habits.** My eating habits are so atrocious, all my other failings are mere peccadillos. As long as I have this terrible weight problem, why bother trying to improve my grooming, dress nicely, stop smoking, control my temper, get off drugs, stop drinking so much, or gamble less? If I licked the weight problem, then I'd have to clean up too many other parts of my act.

☐ **I stay overweight to downplay my other problems.** I'm so fat, my other problems pale by comparison. As long as I have my weight problem to occupy me, I don't have to work on phobias or obsessions or guilt or my relationship with my mother or finishing my degree or getting on with my career or straightening out my finances or finding a decent place to live or dealing with my kids' problems in school. My motto is first things first. (which in this case means first things never.)

☐ **I stay overweight to protect my identity.** I've lost weight before, and it's scary. When I take off a lot of weight quickly, my sense of who I am is threatened. I look in the mirror and don't recognize myself. I don't just lose weight, I lose who I am. I get myself back by regaining the lost pounds.

## What To Do

Now that you've gone through these checklists, what do you do about it?

First, for the "when, where, and what" problems, try applying some of the practical tips offered in this chapter. You'll also find more of these kinds of tips in popular magazines. Truthfully, simple changes of when, where, and what eating behaviors don't contribute much to long-term weight control. Your heredity, metabolism, dieting history, nutrition, exercise, and emotional factors are much more significant in determining your ultimate weight. By the time you've worked through the chapters on improving nutrition and increasing exercise, you will have solved most of your when, where, and what problems. If particular times, places, or foods are still big problems, there are several special sections to handle them in the last chapter on sticking with your program over the long term.

Second, the next chapter shows you how to clean up *why* you eat. The basic idea is to satisfy nutritional needs with food and emotional needs with something more appropriate than food, such as companionship, love, play, reassurance, and so on.

Third, if you have uncovered some significant reasons for *staying* overweight, reading the rest of this book might not be the best plan for you. You may have other work to do before you can successfully apply the principles of lifetime weight control.

For example, you might need some time to figure out how to preserve the important feeling of being "big" without having to be fat. Writing in a diary or talking with a friend might help you explore ways of setting comfortable limits and boundaries made of something other than flesh.

There are several good self- help books that can help you learn to form new relationships, pursue career goals, manage your time, communicate better, improve grooming, and acquire other skills that are beyond the scope of this book. A therapist or other helping professional might be just what you need to help you resolve emotional problems, cope with fear, change undesired behavior, and so on.

On the other hand, perhaps the mere act of recognizing that you have some reason to stay overweight is sufficient to free you from that reason. If so, you're ready to continue your weight control program.

# 4

# Satisfy Emotional Needs Directly

Have you ever ripped the hem out of a favorite skirt and fixed it with safety pins or staples? Did you ever lose one of the tiny screws out of the hinge of your eyeglasses and replace it with a straight pin? Or use a coat hanger for a radio antenna on your car after some dumb kids ripped off the more conventional aerial? Everybody makes these kinds of makeshift substitutions. You can't find a pen or pencil, so you make out the shopping list with an eyebrow pencil or one of your kid's crayons. You go to make your favorite muffin recipe and you're out of butter and buttermilk, so you use shortening and skim milk with a squeeze of lemon instead.

All these makeshifts work, after a fashion and for a time. Just as eating a package of Hostess® cupcakes will work to make you feel less depressed about your job ... after a fashion and for a time. Just as two "man-sized" turkey pot pies and a pint of Rocky Road will help get you through a lonely evening ... after a fashion and for a time.

People who persist in inappropriate, makeshift solutions to life's practical problems are often considered eccentric. They go through life with eyeglasses dangling and rusty coat hangers flopping in the wind, leaving a trail of bent staples, crayon stubs, and unappetizing muffins. Sometimes they're geniuses. Sometimes they're amusing. Often they're neither.

If you persist in solving emotional problems inappropriately by overeating, you can become an emotional eccentric. After years of confusing food with love, hope, diversion, courage, and solace, you can end up with a weight problem on top of the unfulfilled emotional needs you started with.

Filling your emotional needs with food is a very short-term solution. Just as a ripped hem ultimately needs a line of basting stitches, job depression will never really lift until you find a new line of work. Like your radio that will never get good reception without a proper antenna, your love life will never flourish until you learn to take care of yourself as well as your lover.

## Being Happy Is Harder Than Being Thin

Filling emotional needs appropriately with something besides food is very difficult, for several reasons. First of all, the pursuit of food is just plain easier than the pursuit of happiness. When you're under stress, it's easier to order a pizza than it is to take a walk or do a relaxation exercise. When you're lonely, it's easier to raid the icebox than it is to pick up the telephone and find someone to visit. When you're angry at your husband for spending too much money, it's easier to take an extra helping of moussaka than it is to bring up the explosive topic of a family budget.

Second, it's difficult to break the habits of a lifetime. You've been eating your way out of the blues since you were thirteen. You've been making courage out of chocolate milk since you went out for cheerleader in junior high. Cheesecake has been your father confessor since Eisenhower was in office. Reaching for the Ruffles® when the bills come due each month has become a ritual, an automatic reaction that's almost biological in its intensity and inevitability.

Third, there's the fear of change. You'll be replacing your old, comfortable habits with untried and unfamiliar behaviors. You'll literally become a different person, and how do you know you'll like being that person? Although you may be unhappy now, at least you know how to be your unhappy self. You may be lonely or afraid, but at least you know the rules of the game. Is the chance of winning future happiness worth the risk of stepping out on a foreign chessboard, where you're unsure of the moves?

Fourth, and finally, consider the related issue of control. You are attempting to give up using food to control anxiety, anger, and depression. You're going to learn how to control painful emotions more directly with stress reduction, assertiveness, coping skills, and so on. Although you're really taking control of your life at a higher level, it's easy to lose sight of that fact and experience the changes as a *loss* of control.

This perceived loss of control comes at a time when you are losing another source of that "in control" feeling: dieting. When you first go on a diet, you feel in control of your life. Later, when you go off the diet and regain weight, that feeling of control proves to be an illusion. But while it lasts, it's a powerful feeling, a rewarding feeling, a feeling you don't want to give up.

When you make a commitment to stop all future dieting, you remove that periodic illusion of being in control. You create a gap in your life, an emptiness, perhaps even the feeling of being helpless, being out of of control. This is especially true if you've been maintaining an artificially low weight and now allow yourself to give into cravings and gain weight. The feeling of being out of control can be overwhelming.

## Controlling Your Weight Means Controlling Your Life

To make lifetime weight control work, you need to gain some real control over your life. You've already started that process by working on self-acceptance in chapter two and by raising your consciousness about your eating habits in the last chapter.

In this chapter you'll gain further control over your life by learning to satisfy emotional needs directly and appropriately instead of indirectly by overeating.

This chapter can't solve all your emotional problems, but it can point the way. It can get you started in the right direction. It can teach the basics: how to relax and reduce stress without overeating, how to plan and reinforce alternate behaviors to replace old eating habits, and how to get the support you need to make important changes in your life.

# Relaxation and Stress Reduction

A lot of unnecessary, impulsive eating is caused by stress. Food has a tremendous calming, soothing effect that offers relief from the demands of daily life.

You can fill your need for relaxation directly by learning short, simple relaxation exercises and doing them instead of heading for the snack bar. It's especially valuable to do relaxation exercises before your main meal of the day. If you come to the table already relaxed and calm, you'll enjoy eating more and be less inclined to wolf down more than you really need.

The best basic relaxation exercises are progressive muscle relaxation and deep breathing.

### Progressive Muscle Relaxation

You can do this exercise lying down on your back or sitting up in a comfortable chair. Start by closing your eyes and uncrossing your arms and legs.

Make a fist with each hand and squeeze tight. Really concentrate on the feeling of tension in your fists and forearms. Raise your arms to the side, in a "Charles Atlas" pose and flex your biceps. Hold this tension for about seven seconds, then let your arms fall limp to your sides.

Focus on the sensations of warmth and heaviness that flood through your arms as you let them flop down, completely limp. Repeat this flexing and releasing another time, really concentrating on the contrast between tension and relaxation in your arms.

All "nervous tension" is really muscular tension. When you feel tense and "stressed out," it's because various muscles in your body are tensed up to help you face some challenge. Progressive muscle relaxation is actually a way of sensitizing yourself to your body's unique patterns of tension.

Now move your awareness to your chest and back. Take a deep breath and hold it. Tense your chest, shoulders, and upper back muscles, making your entire upper torso rigid. After about seven seconds, let out the breath with a long, loud sigh and let your torso go limp. Melt down into the bed or chair and focus on the difference between the tense and relaxed states. Take another breath and repeat the process until the difference is clear.

A lot of people tense their back and shoulder muscles under stress, as if preparing to ward off a blow from behind. This makes it difficult to breathe deeply, depriving your body of oxygen and increasing your stress level.

Now move your attention downward into your stomach, lower back, and pelvic regions. Tighten your stomach, lower back, and buttocks carefully. If you're lying down, raise your knees slightly to take the strain off your back. Don't overdo the tensing in this area or you might throw your back out. After seven seconds, relax and melt again into the bed or chair. Notice the difference between the tension and relaxation. Repeat the tensing and relaxing one more time.

Some people tense their stomach muscles when stress levels go up. This restricts the movement of your diaphragm, making it hard to get a full breath. Breathing becomes shallow and rapid, sometimes leading to hyperventilation and a full-blown panic attack.

Now work on your legs. Tense your thighs, your calves, and your feet. If you have trouble tensing the various muscles in your lower legs, alternately pull your feet up toward your head and then push them them down away from your head. Hold the tension for several seconds, then let your legs totally relax. Feel the heaviness and warmth flood into your legs as they go completely limp. Repeat the sequence one more time.

When you are under stress, your leg muscles can tense up in an unconscious preparation to run away from danger. Since you rarely follow through and actually run away, the unreleased tension in your legs becomes part of that chronic feeling of being under stress, being unable to let go and relax.

The last area to work on is your neck and head. Tense your neck muscles by shrugging your shoulders upward as far as you can, but don't try to pull your neck in like a turtle. At the same time, clench your jaw muscles carefully—no need to bear down hard enough to crack a tooth. Now frown deeply, making your whole face as wrinkled as the meat of a walnut. Then relax and let your shoulders drop, your jaw hang slightly open. Repeat until you can really feel the relaxation in this critical area.

Under stress it's common to hunch your shoulders up, tense your neck muscles, and grind your teeth. The neck, shoulder, and jaw areas are the most common areas in which people store muscular tension.

Now scan back over your entire body and see if there is any residual tension. If you find any areas that remain tense, repeat the muscle tightening and loosening sequence.

The first few times you try progressive relaxation, it will take you as much as ten minutes to go through all your muscle groups, and you may not get completely relaxed. But as you become more familiar with the technique, you will come to recognize the sensations of muscular tension more quickly and be able to release muscular tension rapidly.

You'll also learn where in your body you habitually hold tension, and work on those areas first. Soon you will be able to scan your body and relax at will, with only mild tensing and stretching of the tight spots. You'll find yourself adjusting the progressive muscle relaxation procedures to fit your unique tension patterns.

### Deep Breathing

This is a very simple stress reduction technique you can use any time, any place. Practice it at first lying down. Later you can do it sitting, standing, or even while walking.

Lie down and close your eyes. Place one hand lightly on your stomach and the other hand on your chest. Breathe in slowly, through your nose if possible. Take a full, deep breath into your stomach and watch how the hand on your stomach rises. The hand on your chest should move only slightly or not at all. Pause a moment, then breathe out slowly through your mouth with a soft "whooshing" sound.

The idea is to breathe deeply into the lower part of your lungs, filling them to the very bottom and pushing your stomach up. Just concentrate on breathing into your stomach and you'll soon be doing it easily.

This is "belly breathing." Your diaphragm is moving freely through its complete range. It is literally impossible to breathe like this, slowly and deeply, and feel tense. Deep breathing has a profound relaxing effect on your entire body. It sends a message to your autonomic nervous system that all is well.

To enhance the relaxing effects of deep breathing, you can practice a simple meditation technique called breath counting. When you inhale, say "one" to yourself. When you exhale, say "two." When you inhale again, start over with "one." This simple one-two counting engages your mind in a repetitive task that makes it easier to avoid distracting thoughts. Some people like to repeat a mantra word like "peace" or "calm" with each breath instead of counting. This has essentially the same effect as counting.

Any time you feel uptight and get the urge for a candy bar or a soda, try half a dozen deep breaths. The feeling of nervous hunger will often pass and you'll be able to do without the snack. This technique works even better if you combine the breathing with a walking meditation. Get up and walk around for a minute. Match your slow steps to the rhythm of your breathing and count your steps. The physical action, deep breathing, and counting combine to give you a change of scene, calm and refresh your body, and distract your mind.

## Visualization

Being able to physically relax your body is the first step in using visualization to achieve more profound levels of relaxation. Visualization enhances relaxation by fooling your mind into thinking you are having a very relaxing experience: lying in the sun on the beach, strolling in the woods, or paddling a canoe on a quiet lake.

The visualization that follows is adapted from my book, *Visualization for Change.* You can use it with your own variations to create an imaginary special place that is very relaxing to you, a place that you can return to again and again.

*Visualization*

Lie on your back with your arms and legs un-crossed. Close your eyes and relax using progressive muscle relaxation and breathing.

You are going to gradually create a special place for yourself in nature. The instructions will be necessarily somewhat vague, since you have to fill in details that you find particularly relaxing.

Imagine a path. It can be in the woods, at the seashore, in the desert, or the mountains. It can be a place you know or would like to know. Imagine that you are standing on the path, looking down it. Notice the surface of the path: the color and texture of the dirt, the sand, the rocks. Look at the grass and shrubs on either side. Begin walking on the path and notice how it feels against your feet.

As you stroll down the path, look up and notice the countryside. See the colors and shapes of the trees, rocks, mountains, or whatever. Listen and hear the birds, the sound of water, of wind, and of your own steps. Notice how quiet and peaceful it is here in this special place. Take a deep breath and smell the fresh air. Take in the smells of earth, water, and green growing things. Feel the sun shining and a gentle breeze blowing against your face.

Continue down the path until you come to some sort of enclosed area. This will be your special place. Take a look around this special spot. It can be an area of soft sand on the beach, a clearing in the woods, a meadow on a mountain side, a grassy bank by a stream, or whatever you want. Notice its shape and general layout. Notice the ground, rocks, grass, bushes, and so on. What can you hear, smell, and feel?

Find a comfortable place to lie down. It could be the sun-warmed sand, a bed of dry moss or leaves, a blanket spread on the grass—anywhere you like. Lie on your back and try it out. It's peaceful and serene. You're neither too warm or too cool. You're just comfortable, just floating in pure relaxation.

As you lie there letting the sun soak into you, feel heavier and heavier. Sink down into the sand or grass as you become more and more relaxed.

This is your place, special for you alone. You are safe and secure here. None of your usual worries can touch you here. You can come here any time you want to relax.

Enjoy your special place until you feel completely relaxed. When you're ready to come back, imagine getting up and strolling away from your special place.

Remind yourself of your actual surroundings, open your eyes, and get up slowly. As you go about your daily routine, remember that you have a special place to which you can retreat briefly for rest and renewal.

### Changing Your Lifestyle

Over the long term, the way to beat stress is to change your lifestyle. If you're an air traffic controller or a bullfighter, deep breathing is only going to relieve part of your job stress. If you live with moody, unpredictable, violent people, progressive relaxation is only going to remove a fraction of your anxiety. If you drink six cups of coffee and smoke a pack of cigarettes every day, your stress reduction efforts will be drowned in a flood of stimulants. And even thirty-minute daily meditation or self-hypnosis sessions won't help much if they are crammed into an eighty-hour work week.

Examine your goals, your values, your living arrangements, and your schedule. Figure out what's really important to you. Look for sources of stress that can be cut out, cut back, or avoided. Consider changing your job or your living arrangements. By reducing the demands on your time and resources, you can cut the number of stressors to which you must respond. That's real stress reduction.

## Plan Alternative Behaviors

You need to plan exactly what you are going to do instead of eating when you start feeling sad, bored, anxious, and so on. As soon as a familiar feeling like boredom steals over you and you think about getting something to eat, you will instead remember your planned alternative behavior and go for a walk or work on your knitting. When you realize that you're nervous about an upcoming appointment, that will be your signal to do five minutes of progressive muscle relaxation instead of making some toast and tea.

Take a look at your "why I eat" checklist from the previous chapter. In that checklist you began to identify feelings that often trigger your inappropriate eating. Now you will expand this information and use it as a guide for planning alternative behaviors.

Read carefully through the following list and check off or underline the feelings that trigger eating for you, the real needs that you seem to be trying to meet, and any of the suggested alternative behaviors that appeal to you. Use the extra spaces to add alternative behaviors better suited to your individual interests, situation, and abilities.

| Feelings that Trigger Eating | Real Needs | Alternative Behaviors To Meet Needs |
|---|---|---|
| lonely<br>alone<br>abandoned | companionship<br>belonging<br>inclusion | call a friend<br>visit somebody<br>get a pet<br>go to a club meeting<br>take a class<br>go to singles group<br><br>—————————<br>—————————  |
| sad<br>depressed<br>sense of loss<br>hopeless<br>nervous | happiness<br>hope<br>meaning | tell best friend about it<br>go jogging<br>work on strength list<br>do visualization exercise<br><br>—————————<br>—————————  |
| anxious<br>scared<br>frightened<br>nervous | relaxation<br>stress reduction<br>safety | progressive muscle<br>    relaxation<br>deep breathing<br>share feelings with<br>    someone<br>analyze and refute my<br>    catastrophic thinking<br><br>—————————<br>—————————  |
| bored<br>restless | activity<br>interest | practice piano<br>juggling<br>take a walk<br>rearrange furniture,<br>    desk, kitchen drawers<br>go to a movie<br>rent a video<br><br>—————————<br>—————————  |
| tired<br>fatigued<br>worn out | rest<br>relaxation | take a nap<br>meditate<br>postpone commitments<br><br>—————————<br>—————————  |

| Feelings that Trigger Eating | Real Needs | Alternative Behaviors To Meet Needs |
|---|---|---|
| deserving<br>lacking<br>empty | reward<br>acknow-<br>ledgement<br>to be filled up | take a trip to the hobby<br>store<br>buy some flowers for<br>myself<br>review past successes<br>have my hair done at the<br>expensive salon<br>buy the hardcover<br>instead of waiting for<br>the paperback<br><br>_____<br>_____ |
| angry<br>resentful<br>frustrated<br>jealous | to be heard<br>assert my rights<br>revenge<br>hit something | use problem solving<br>together<br>fill out<br>"think/feel/want"<br>form from assertive-<br>ness workshop<br>hit a pillow<br>confront my lover with<br>my suspicions<br><br>_____<br>_____ |
| unloved<br>unworthy | self-worth<br>to be loved<br>re-experience<br>mother's love | hug someone<br>cuddle and kiss<br>tell someone "I love you"<br>make love<br>use self-acceptance -<br>affirmations<br>call mom<br><br>_____<br>_____ |

| Feelings that Trigger Eating | Real Needs | Alternative Behaviors To Meet Needs |
|---|---|---|
| guilty<br>bad<br>wrong<br>undeserving | forgiveness<br>atonement<br>punishment | refute guilty thoughts<br>use "I'm only human/I<br>  forgive myself"<br>  affirmations<br>donate money to charity<br>do volunteer work<br>tell myself that past<br>  actions are over and<br>  done with<br><br>_____<br><br>_____ |
| oppressed<br>discriminated<br>  against<br>in the minority | equality<br>assert my rights<br>revenge | join support group<br>write a letter to my<br>  congressperson<br>talk it over with a like-<br>  minded friend<br>speak up to challenge<br>  sexism and fatism<br><br>_____<br><br>_____ |
| happy<br>proud<br>sense of<br>  accomplish-<br>  ment<br>relieved some-<br>  thing's over | celebration<br>reward | buy myself a present<br>listen to favorite music<br>go out dancing<br><br>_____<br><br>_____ |
| shy<br>tongue-tied<br>bashful<br>socially inept | confidence<br>make contact | practice coping<br>  statements<br>use prepared opening<br>  lines<br>keep occupied at parties<br>  helping or dancing<br><br>_____<br><br>_____ |

| Feelings that Trigger Eating | Real Needs | Alternative Behaviors To Meet Needs |
|---|---|---|
| hurt | recognition | tell about my hurt without blaming |
| mistreated | appreciation | |
| unappreciated | _____ | ask for what I want assertively |
| _____ | _____ | write in my journal to clarify what hurts |
| | | _____ |
| | | _____ |
| _____ | _____ | _____ |
| _____ | _____ | _____ |
| | | _____ |
| _____ | _____ | _____ |
| _____ | _____ | _____ |
| | | _____ |

Spend plenty of time on this exercise, until you have clearly identified the feelings that drive you toward food, the real needs you are trying to fill, and some good alternative behaviors you can perform to fill these needs. Use this list to make up affirmation cards in this format:

When I feel ___(feeling that triggers eating)___ ,
I fill my need for____(real need)____
by ___(alternative behavior)___
or ___(second alternative behavior)___
instead of eating.

Be as specific as possible in describing what you will do. Instead of writing "go for a walk," write "walk up to the railroad tracks and see if the willows have budded yet." Instead of just planning to review your strengths the next time you're feeling unworthy, plan to think of five times in the past when you demonstrated compassion and kindness. Also, notice that you should have at least two alternative behaviors planned, to increase your options and be prepared for different circumstances.

Here are some effective alternative behavior plans as they would be written on affirmation cards:

When I feel *lonely*
I fill my need for *companionship*
by *calling up Bill to go to coffee*
or *going next door to chat with Rita*
instead of eating.

When I feel *anxious about my relationship with Barry*
I fill my need for *reassurance*
by *telling him exactly how I'm feeling at the moment*
or *doing a receptive meditation to explore my feelings*
instead of eating.

When I feel *bored and restless*
I fill my need for *activity*
by *going to the library to browse*
or *repotting the bulbs in the greenhouse*
instead of eating.

When I feel *like I deserve a treat*
I fill my need for *a reward*
by *listening to opera*
or *ordering that cross-stitch pattern from the craft catalog*
instead of eating.

When I feel *I need love*
I fill my need for *contact*
by *reaching for Don*
or *hugging one of the kids*
instead of eating chocolate.

Use these affirmations the way you did the affirmations in the chapter on self-acceptance: choose the feelings that bother you most and write your affirmations on two or three cards a day. Carry the cards with you at all times and read them to yourself and aloud every hour. Record your statements on a loop tape. Write them out in the form of a three-column self-dialogue. Post your cards, self-stick notes, or stickers where you will see them often and be reminded of your plans for emotional self-care. Use active integration by writing down examples of times in the past when you met your emotional needs appropriately.

Every time you feel like falling into your old patterns of eating to relieve boredom or depression or whatever, repeat the appropriate affirmation to yourself. You may still decide to eat the brownie or the hot dog, but mentally recite the affirmation anyway. Eventually you'll be able to perform some of your alternate behaviors instead of eating.

Avoid turning these plans into "from now on," absolute resolutions. That way lies madness. That way lies the same obsessive, make-it-or-break-it dieting attitude that you are trying to escape. It has taken you all your life to form your eating habits. It will probably take you a considerable amount of time to change those habits. Treat your plans for alternative behaviors as statements of long-term intention. Just remembering your plan at the appropriate time is a success, even if you don't perform the alternate behavior. Allow your affirmations the time they need to reprogram your unconscious.

Make up different affirmation cards every few days. Over time, some of your affirmations will lose their power to inspire. Then it's time to make up new ones, incorporating new alternate behaviors to match your changing circumstances.

### Dealing with Negative Thoughts

During the process of working on your alternative behavior plans, you may have recurring negative thoughts and predictions: "This will never work ... I'm wasting my time ... This is stupid ... Hopeless," and so on. These self-statements can come to you very quickly, seemingly out of nowhere. They can be gone in an instant, yet leave you completely depressed and demoralized.

If this happens, spend some time bringing these thoughts out into the open. Allow yourself to dwell on the negative thoughts for a while. Really wallow in them. Try to slow the statements down and extract the full text of your mental monologue. For example, the single word "hopeless," coupled with an image of a fat old man you once saw in a nursing home, may be your own mental shorthand for this prediction: "It's hopeless to try to control my weight. I'm going to die a fat person."

When you have clearly identified the negative thoughts that are keeping you stuck, refer back to the chapters on handling fears and improving self-acceptance. Use the hopes and fears exercise and the affirmation techniques taught there to analyze your negative thoughts, refute them, and replace them with positive self-statements.

### Alternative Behavior Exercise

Visualization is a way of using your imagination to bring about your desired behavior changes. You create carefully plotted mental movies of yourself successfully performing your alternative behaviors instead of filling emotional needs with food. This self-image counters and gradually replaces your old self-image of yourself as a person with a weight problem.

To do the exercise, lie down on your back and close your eyes. Take a minute to relax. Use the progressive muscle technique, deep breathing, or any other relaxation technique that works for you.

First imagine that you are in your home. In your mind's eye, recreate the sights and sounds, the textures, smells, and tastes of home: how the sunlight falls across the fruit bowl in the morning, the hat rack in the hall, the corner of the couch that's frayed where the cat sharpens her claws, the sound of the clock on the wall, the distant traffic, the smell of coffee and spices in the kitchen, the feel of your toothbrush, the taste of water from the tap. Make the scene as real and vivid as you can.

Pick one of the problem feelings that you're working on. For example, imagine that you're sitting around your apartment after work, feeling depressed and hungry. Really feel that hunger, that urge to lighten your mood with a peanut butter and jelly and cream cheese sandwich. Use details from your own life: how you usually feel, what you usually crave.

Now listen to yourself repeat an affirmation out loud. For instance: "When I feel restless, I work on my current art project instead of eating."

Now form an intense image of yourself performing your alternative behavior. See yourself going to the back porch and getting down your paint box or your half-finished airplane model. Watch yourself starting to work on something creative—slowly and disinterestedly at first, but with growing interest and enjoyment.

Feel the hunger fade, replaced by a glow of achievement and self-satisfaction. Congratulate yourself: "I'm really doing it. I'm fighting boredom and depression by mobilizing myself into action."

Repeat the scene, using another alternative behavior. See yourself inviting someone over to watch a video with you, or going for a walk, or taking a bubble bath—whatever new, alternative behaviors you are trying out. Include positive self-statements and the feeling of accomplishment and well being.

For future visualization sessions, change the scene to a restaurant, your mom's house, or an office party—wherever your problem feelings crop up. See yourself successfully initiating and carrying out your alternative behavior.

Do these visualizations at least once a day. More often is better. You can even do short, ten-second scenes while you're riding on the bus, drying your hair, or waiting for your toast to pop up.

As with the affirmations, some scenes will eventually lose interest and vividness. You'll have to make up new ones as you go along. After a while, you'll notice that your alternative behaviors seem easier to do in real life. They'll feel more natural and you'll actually start to enjoy them for their own sake.

## Get Support

You can get some of your emotional needs met on your own, but that's doing it the hard way. Getting your emotional needs met— and indeed your whole program of lifetime weight control—will go much easier and faster when you have the active support of family, friends, and lovers.

Support from others comes in many forms. Really supportive people know what you are trying to do, are willing to try more nutritious foods with you, join you in physical activities, congratulate your successes, help get back on track after setbacks, and so on.

Don't just ask your spouse or your best friend to "support" you and let it go at that. Discuss in detail what you want them to do for you and with you. A good way to do this is to make a photocopy of the following support agreement and go over it with them line by line. Cross out what doesn't apply to you. Add additional kinds of support you want. Do this with each significant person in your life, the ones whose support will be crucial to your success.

If it seems too weird or corny to be signing agreements with your mother, your lover, or whoever, at least show them this part of the book. Say "I'd really like your help in this new program I'm trying, and here's a good list of ways you might help me."

SUPPORT AGREEMENT

I, _____

agree to help you,_____

in your program of lifetime weight control.

To the best of my ability, I will:

Help you meet your emotional needs appropriately.

Take you seriously, without condescension.

Accept you just the way you are.

Not criticize you or anyone else for being overweight.

Not talk about or encourage dieting in any way.

Compliment you on your determination.

Regularly check in with you about your progress.
Congratulate you on your successes.
Notice and comment when you look better.
Notice and comment when you seem to feel better.
Remind you of your goals when you forget.
Encourage you when you get discouraged.
Console you during setbacks.
Defend your efforts when talking to others.
Learn more about lifetime weight control.
Suspend judgment if I disagree with something you're trying.
Keep my doubts to myself.
Make only constructive suggestions.
Learn more about nutrition with you.
Help you shop for more nutritious foods.
Help you cook more nutritious foods.
Join you in eating more nutritious foods such as

_____.

Let you eat what you want, without criticism.
Not tempt you with unhealthy foods such as

_____.

Not eat junk food in front of you.
Join you in physical activities such as

_____.

Watch your kids so you can go to a dance or exercise class.
Not kid you about the affirmation file cards and signs.

_____

_____

_____

_____


_____
(signature)

*Other Kinds of Support*

Support is just a trendy word for help, and help can come from many sources. Self-help books, community college classes, workshops, clubs, support groups, and therapists are good sources of help for ending loneliness, lifting depression, coping with fears, and building self-esteem.

If you eat to express resentment, try assertiveness training instead. If you eat whenever you have discipline problems with your kids, try a parenting workshop instead.

Help is out there, waiting for you to seek it. Take the energy you used to put into dieting and agonizing about your weight and invest it in your own growth.

If you decide to see a therapist or join a weight control support group, take care. Make sure that the individuals you turn to know that traditional dieting is a trap. Make sure they will support your program of lifetime weight control.

# 5

# Improve Nutrition

You can overeat, be overweight, and still be undernourished. If you've been dieting off and on for years,
you probably live in a state of chronic, subclinical
malnutrition. Even when you're consuming lots of
calories, you may not be getting the right balance of
the forty to sixty nutrients you need to stay healthy.

Because your malnutrition is subclinical, you
don't have any obvious symptoms like skin erup-
tions or rickets. You are just easily tired, susceptible
to colds and flu, bowled over by stress, easily
angered, or prone to depression or anxiety. And because your condition is chronic, you don't really
know what it feels like to be in peak health. Dragging
around feels "normal" to you.

This chapter will help you begin to switch your
focus: from your appearance to your health, from
how you look to how you feel, from food choices
based on calories and cravings to food choices based
on nutrition and a healthy appetite.

## The Curse of Calorie Consciousness

Is this you? You're walking down the street and see a kid eating an ice cream cone and automatically think "five hundred calories." You look at a small pork chop in the meat counter and catch yourself calculating its weight in grams. You bite into an apple fritter and there comes unbidden to your mind a vision of the roll of flab that sticks out over the top of your bathing suit.

This is the dieter's way of thinking about food: in terms of calories and amounts and how fat it can make you.

Improving your nutrition starts with changing your automatic thoughts about food. You need to stop thinking in the short term about calories and weight and start thinking in the long term about nutrition and health. You need to switch your focus from your appearance in the mirror today to your health and vigor five or ten years from now.

But what about the "stop dieting" rule? What about eating spontaneously? How can you eat spontaneously, choosing whatever you feel like eating, and still improve your nutrition?

Good question. At first you can't do both. At first, it's more important to eat whenever you feel hungry and to eat whatever appeals to you. Breaking your chronic dieter's hangups about "good" food and "bad" food is more important in the beginning than nutritional considerations.

That's why "eat spontaneously" is the first step in lifetime weight control and "improve nutrition" is the fifth step. However, you can eventually reconcile spontaneous eating with choosing more nutritious foods. Once you have learned to eat spontaneously, you will seldom crave specific foods. Most of the time, you'll just be hungry in general, and many different types of food will satisfy you. When you reach that point, you'll have the latitude to choose nutritious foods and still be eating spontaneously.

## The Curse of Abundance

Your mind may be living in the twentieth century, but your body is that of a cave dweller. In prehistoric times, food was often scarce. The early humans who survived were the ones with a strong hunger drive, the ones who were good at finding and consuming food. They had a built-in craving for high-energy foods like animal fat and honey—concentrated food sources that could keep them going for a long time.

The human appetite evolved over millions of years in conditions of scarcity that do not obtain today. Today the food environment is cursed with abundance. Everywhere you look, fatty, sugary foods are readily available. And your prehistoric appetite wants you to eat them. It will be thousands of years, if ever, before the slow forces of evolution produce a human race with an appetite geared for abundance.

In the meantime, you have to educate yourself about nutrition in order to avoid the hidden fats, sugars, salts, and so on that surround you.

## Guidelines to Better Nutrition

TV shows, magazine articles, and books giving nutritional advice abound. So much information can become very confusing. Nutrition is such a vast subject that you can find yourself overwhelmed. It can seem as if eating "correctly" requires a doctorate in biology.

For that reason, I'm going to keep this section as simple and clear as possible. The most important guideline comes first, the second most important guideline comes second, and so on. Follow these guidelines in sequence and you can be sure that you are improving your nutrition as quickly and effectively as possible.

Read the first section on eating a variety of foods and then stop reading. Work on adding variety to your diet first and don't worry about fat or sugar or salt. Making one kind of change in your eating habits at a time is all you can reasonably expect yourself to do. If you try to revolutionize your complete diet all at once, you're probably doomed to failure. Your food preferences are habits you've taken a lifetime to acquire. You can't change them overnight.

Give yourself at least three months to put each guideline into effect. You need at least that much time to get used to the changes in your diet and let your natural cravings subside.

And don't worry if you backslide. Personal change is seldom a straight-line path to a goal. You can expect some setbacks, some reversals, and some "resting" periods in which you abandon your eating goals and focus on something else in your life. Remember, you're taking the long view now: your hip and waist measurements next summer are irrelevant—now you're focusing on your continued feelings of health and vitality for the rest of your life.

## 1. Eat a Variety of Foods

To stay healthy, you need a wide variety of nutrients: forty to sixty different vitamins, minerals, essential fatty acids, amino acids, trace elements, fats, proteins, carbohydrates. The list goes on and on.

Most foods contain more than one essential nutrient, but there is no single, perfect food. Milk was touted for years by the dairy industry as "nature's most nearly perfect food," and it's true that milk does provide proteins, sugars, fats, B vitamins, vitamin A, calcium, and phosphorus. However, milk is a lousy source of iron or vitamin C, and millions of people in the world lack the digestive bacteria necessary to properly digest milk.

Every year scientists discover another vitamin or trace element that plays an important, previously unknown role in human nutrition. The vitamin supplement manufacturers duly jump on the bandwagon and add the new miracle nutrient to their line of capsules and tablets.

But food is still the major and most important source of all the known—and unknown—nutrients that you need to thrive. And the single best thing you can do to improve your nutrition is to eat a wide variety of foods. The more variety in your diet, the more likely you are to get all the nutrients you need. Variety will also reduce the likelihood of being exposed to a lot of contaminants in any one kind of food.

The best way to add variety to your diet is to do what they told you in grammar school and high school: eat something every day from each of the four major food groups:

| FOOD GROUP | SERVINGS PER DAY |
|---|---|
| Vegetables and fruits | 4 |
| Bread, cereal, grain products | 4 |
| Meat, poultry, fish, eggs, beans, peas | 2 |
| Milk, cheese, yogurt | 2 |
| | (3 or 4 for teens, pregnant women and nursing mothers) |

Remember the three-by-five cards you used to keep track of what you ate for a week? Look them over again and see which of these food groups you eat too much of and which you avoid. If you're like most people, you eat a lot of meat and not as much from the vegetables and fruits group.

Think of this step toward better nutrition as *adding variety*, not *removing* foods you like. At this stage, don't say to yourself, "I'll have fruit instead of bacon for breakfast." Rather, say "I'll have fruit *as well as* bacon."

Start with one or two specific foods that you want to add first. Figure out how you'll get these foods and when you'll eat them. Here are some suggestions.

- Order a salad to go with your pizza.
- Buy a different kind of bread at the market.
- Share entrees at restaurants.
- Scan menus for dishes you've never tried.
- Buy exotic fruits instead of the usual apples and oranges.
- Go to a health food store and browse for things you've never tried.
- Use parsnips as well as carrots in stew.
- Sample different kinds of yogurt and cheese.

When you're selecting different kinds of food that you don't usually eat, you can try to pick low fat items, or whole foods rather than processed foods. But don't worry too much about those aspects. The important thing is to eat a lot of different kinds of food and find new things that you like to eat.

You'll have better nutrition, better weight control, and an easier time increasing variety if you eat three or four small meals a day. It's better for your body and less fattening to eat three small meals than it is to eat the same total amount of food at one big meal. Don't kid yourself that skipping meals is a good way to control weight. Skipping meals will make you eat *more* in the long run. Your body will sense that there is some kind of food shortage, and compensate by increasing your appetite to make sure you eat lots of food when you do eat. Over time, you'll drift into the high end of your setpoint weight range.

Breakfast and lunch are the meals people skip most often. Shop for a week's worth of breakfasts and lunches. Pick foods that are nutritious, easy to prepare, and easy to take to work or school. If you have the foods on hand and have a plan to eat them, you'll be less likely to skip meals or grab junk food snacks on the run.

To educate yourself about the wide variety of food choices open to you, wander through a big supermarket and look at all the things you've never tried. Also browse in a health food store to discover new things to eat and healthy alternatives to some of your old favorite junk foods. While you're there, pick up a "healthy foods" cookbook and some information on nutrition.

Work your new food choices into the visualization and affirmation excercises that the previous chapters introduced. After a relaxation exercise, visualize yourself snacking on whole wheat bread and cream cheese instead of your usual Ritz® and cheddar. Tell yourself, "I like lots of different, nutritious foods." If you are taping up three-by-five cards with affirmations on them, include a couple that say, "When I go to a restaurant, I look for something different," or "At George's I can have nuts or popcorn as well as the usual cold cuts," or "I eat to maintain health, not my figure."

## 2. Reduce Fat

Don't try to put this guideline into action until you have worked on increasing variety for at least three months. By that time you will have a good idea of what foods are available to you and which ones you like. Then you can start evaluating foods for their fat content.

To stay healthy, about thirty percent of your total diet should be made up of fats. But the average person eats way too much fat—closer to forty-five percent.

There are three kinds of fat:

**1. Saturated fat** tends to be solid at room temperature. It's found in all meats, lard, hydrogenated shortening, coconut oil, palm oil, dairy products, and chocolate. This is the worse kind of fat you can eat. Although there is some controversy about how fats, cholesterol, blood pressure, and heart disease are related, the most widely accepted theory suggests that saturated fats raise the amount of cholesterol in your blood, which can lead to heart disease.

Saturated fat is insidious. It's present in all sorts of products like cakes, pastries, cookies, gravy, non-dairy creamers, candy, sauces, and many snack foods.

**2. Monosaturated fat** tends to be liquid at room temperature but solidifies when chilled. Examples are olive oil, peanut oil, avocados, and most nuts. These foods are a little better for you than the saturated fats.

**3. Polyunsaturated fat** stays liquid even when chilled. Oils made from safflower, corn, soybeans, and cottonseed contain polyunsaturated fats. Other foods containing polyunsaturated fat are margarine, salad dressings, mayonnaise, walnuts, sesame seeds, and sunflower seeds. These are the safest fats to consume.

If you're worried about your fat intake, have a series of blood tests done to establish your cholesterol level. This is especially important if you smoke or have high blood pressure.

So what do you do to reduce fat in your diet? First, become aware of the fat you eat. Pay attention to the ingredients listed on all the processed food you buy. Start thinking of ways to consume less fat in general, switch to more polyunsaturated fats, and choose food products made with less fat.

Repeat the food diary exercise with the three-by-five cards. You have increased the variety in your diet by now, and you need some new cards to look at. This time, look for high fat foods that you eat a lot of.

Plan to reduce fat over the next three months. For the first month, target the two biggest "fat offenders" in your diet—ice cream, french fries, blue cheese dressing, or whatever. Pick a dish that you eat at restaurants and one that you eat frequently at home. For each high fat dish, pick a low fat substitute that you enjoy. The substitutes can be direct replacements, such as frozen yogurt for ice cream, or just alternative foods that you enjoy, like carrot salad instead of french fries at your favorite cafe. Resolve to make these two substitutions consistently over the next thirty days.

For the second month, pick the two "next worst" high fat foods you usually eat and replace them with low fat foods. Try altering some foods rather than replacing them. For example, if you love making fried chicken, try removing the skin from the chicken pieces before you bread and fry them. It's almost as good, and much lower in fat without the skin. Or broil the chicken with the skin on and then remove it before serving.

Here are some additional ideas for ways to reduce fat in your diet.

• Trim the fat from steaks and chops before cooking or eating.

• Switch from butter to margarine, and put less on your bread, noodles, or potatoes. Many kinds of bread taste delicious with nothing on them.

• Switch from ice cream to nonfat frozen yogurt.

• Bake and broil foods instead of frying them in grease.

• Order clear broth soups instead of creamy ones.

• Buy low fat salad dressings or just use lemon juice.

• Have fish or turkey instead of sausages or pork chops.

• Switch to safflower or corn oil.

• Cut back on fast foods and pastries, which are laced with hidden fats.

In the third month you will replace or modify two more of your favorite high fat foods. After three months, you will have significantly reduced the amount of fat in your diet.

One of the best ways to avoid high fat foods is not to let them into the house in the first place. Good nutrition starts in the grocery store. To maximize the probability of buying nutritious foods, always make a shopping list and don't shop when you're hungry. Take the time before shopping to write down a complete list of everything that you want to buy. Figure out your menus ahead of time and plan to pick up nutritious snacks. When you're writing your list, think in terms of picking foods from all four food groups, picking alternatives to high fat foods, avoiding sugary and salty foods, and so on. This way you'll avoid some of those impulses to fill your cart with whatever looks appealing at the moment.

Shopping when you're hungry just makes it that much harder to resist fatty, sugary foods. If you must shop when you're hungry, then making out a list and sticking to it are even more important.

Get support for your nutritional goals. It's hard to change your eating habits on your own, without the support of the people you live with. It takes incredible moral courage to fix yourself a brown rice casserole when your husband is eating porkchops and fried potatoes with pan gravy. Your oat bran cereal and fresh fruit looks pretty dull when the rest of the family is downing cinnamon rolls and bacon.

If you possibly can, make the switch to better nutrition a family affair. At least get your household to meet you halfway by agreeing to try a new, "good for you" dish each week.

If your family insists on having donuts and potato chips and candy in the house, at least hide these goodies away where you won't have to see them and be tempted. Put them in the back of the crisper drawer or behind the bread box. Hide them on the top shelf of the cupboard. Make your kids keep their junky snacks in their own rooms.

When doing relaxation exercises or weight control visualizations, include some images and suggestions regarding fat reduction. Tell yourself, "I am cutting down on unhealthy fats. I enjoy eating low fat foods." Incorporate images of yourself in the grocery store, in your kitchen, at dinner parties, and at restaurants—chosing lower fat foods and enjoying them mightily.

Is this easy? No. This is a hard step, much harder than the first guideline, which merely asked you to add variety. Here you are having to remove some things you love to eat. The replacements won't taste as good to you. And you're not making these changes just until you lose ten pounds—it's for life.

That's the bad news. The good news is that eventually you will come to prefer bread without butter. Steak fat will eventually taste bad to you. You'll find that whole milk tastes weird once you've gotten used to nonfat milk.

Until that time, give yourself some slack. Allow yourself to indulge in a high fat treat once a week or so. Remind yourself that weight control is a long-term effort. It's the sum total of your food choices over years and years that counts, not whether you have a Polish sausage or a milkshake today.

### 3. Reduce Sugar

Sugar—whether white sugar, brown sugar, honey, molasses, maple syrup, or whatever—is a highly refined product. It is a simple carbohydrate that contains no starch, no fiber, and no vitamins or minerals.

Nutritionally, all you get from sugar is a lot of empty calories that your body must burn up very quickly or rapidly turn into fat.

Fully 25 percent of the calories in the average American diet come from sugar. This amounts to 160 pounds of sugar per adult per year. Cutting down on this huge load of sugar is especially important if you are under stress or are predisposed to diabetes or hypoglycemia. All three of these conditions make you extremely sensitive to variations in your blood sugar level. As your blood sugar level goes up and down, you can experience fluctuations in your energy level, dizzinesss, anxiety, depression, irritability, tremor, nausea, or hunger pangs.

Get out your old three-by-five food diary cards or make a new set by doing the exercise again for a week. Take a look at the sweet things you love most. Pick a sweet that you like to eat out and one that you tend to eat a lot of at home. These are your targets for the next month. Plan what you will eat instead of these two favorites. For example, resolve to order just coffee instead of coffee and cheese cake. Or have fresh fruit for dessert at home instead of ice cream.

After a month, pick two more food items high in sugar and replace them. Instead of Milk Duds® at the movies, get popcorn without butter. Instead of snacking on cookies with your kids in the afternoon, try celery sticks with peanut butter.

From a weight control point of view, there isn't much difference between highly refined sugars like table sugar or corn syrup and more "natural" sweeteners like fruit sugars and honey. But the more natural sugars may be a little more digestible and less likely to be contaminated during the refining process.

Give your sugar reduction efforts at least another month, targeting another two food items. When you're shopping, pick the canned fruit packed in water instead of the stuff in syrup. Buy the low sugar, high fiber cereals instead of the sugar-coated kind.

Get in the habit of looking at labels when you shop. Educate yourself in the many names for sugar and be a little suspicious when you read labels. Processed food products are high in sugar if the first or second ingredient listed is sucrose, glucose, maltose, dextrose, lactose, fructose, or any kind of syrup.

Again, get all the support you can for your anti-sugar campaign. Discourage friends and relatives from giving you food gifts at holiday time. When they give you the box of See's® Nuts and Chews anyway, thank them and tuck the box away. As soon as they're gone, throw it away or wrap it up again and give it to somebody else.

Find someone, friend or relative or advisor, to whom you can talk about your struggles to achieve better nutrition. Make a formal pact with this person: that you will only have dessert on Saturday nights at your mother's, and not any other time. Ask your support person to check in with you periodically to see how you're doing. Promise to acknowledge if you slip, and renew your contract at regular intervals. Your pact will work best if the other person is also working on nutritional goals, and you can make mutual agreements and hold each other to them.

When you do the visualization and relaxation exercises associated with other parts of this book, throw in some images and affirmations about sugar. See yourself refusing dessert. Envision yourself as the kind of person who can take sweets or leave them.

Tell yourself, "I am cutting down on sugar ... I love my body ... I can live without sweets just fine."

Try this special visualization: before you fall asleep at night and just after you wake up in the morning, imagine that you can see a switch inside your head. It's a red plastic pushbutton that is lit up with a harsh glaring light. Imagine that this is the switch that controls your cravings for sweets. Reach out your imaginary finger and push the button to turn it off. See it go dark. Next, visualize an elegant ivory button in a beautiful mahogany control panel. This is the switch that controls your healthy appetite for nutritious foods. Turn it on and see it softly gleam.

If you find the prospect of cutting out sugary treats too daunting, allow yourself an ice cream sundae or a sticky bun on Wednesday mornings, with certain friends, or in a certain restaurant. Deliberately plan when and where and with whom you'll indulge in your favorite treat and really enjoy every moment of eating it.

### Avoid Alcohol

Alcohol is high in calories, low in other nutrients, and tends to stimulate your appetite so that you eat more of other foods. It also depletes your body of the B vitamins, which help you cope with stress.

Many people find it easier to quit alcohol entirely than to cut back to a moderate consumption. What they say in Alcoholics Anonymous is correct: for many people, one drink is too many, because it inevitably leads to excess. If you're going to drink at all, confine your intake to one or two glasses of beer or wine a day and leave the hard stuff alone.

This can be one of the most difficult changes to make in your life. I'd need to write another book just on the subject of drinking alone to give it justice. Here are a few bare-minimum suggestions:

**1. Get support.** This is the foundation of Alcoholics Anonymous— the support of other recovering drinkers. Find someone whom you can call on day or night to help you cut back or stop. Make a formal agreement, written down and signed, about your drinking goals. Check in with your support person regularly, even if you're doing well.

**2. Determine exactly when, where, and how much you'll drink.** And stick to it. This is one instance in which a traditional dieting approach makes sense. If you can stick to your plan consistently, you're probably a social drinker who can enjoy alcohol while maintaining lifetime weight control. Give this step three months of trial, just like the rest of the nutritional guidelines in this chapter. Include alcohol moderation in your visualizations and affirmations.

**3. If moderation doesn't work, quit entirely.** You plan to have just two glasses of wine with dinner, but you have five. You swear off the lunchtime beer but you can't resist. You say you're not going to stop off at the bar after work, but you find yourself there anyway. These are danger signals. They indicate a potential problem with alcohol that goes beyond considerations of weight control. The sooner you quit drinking, the better.

*Eat More Whole Foods*

What are "whole foods"? They are raw or lightly steamed vegetables, fruits, whole wheat products, whole rolled oats, cornmeal, brown rice, beans, dried peas, nuts, and seeds. These are complex carbohydrates containing a healthy mix of fiber, starch, sugar, vitamins, and minerals.

You've already added variety to your diet and cut back on fats and sugar. Inevitably, you have discovered some whole foods that make great replacements for fatty, sugary prepared foods. Now increase your alternatives by actively seeking out whole foods.

Have raw carrot sticks instead of cooked carrots with honey glaze. Have a fresh green salad instead of macaroni or potato salad. Buy whole wheat bread instead of white bread and buy brown rice instead of white rice. Have oatmeal in the morning instead of sugar-coated cereal. Eat fresh fruit instead of canned or processed fruit products.

As with the previous steps, give yourself three months to work on increasing the percentage of whole foods in your diet. Work images of this change into your visualization and relaxation exercises.

### Reduce Sodium

Sodium is an essential nutrient, but the average adult consumes about fifty grams a day—ten times the five grams per day that is required for good health. High sodium intake is associated with high blood pressure, so it is especially important to avoid sodium if you are prone to hypertension.

Sodium is everywhere. Table salt is forty percent sodium. High sodium levels provide the savor in many processed sauces and condiments like pickles, ketchup, potato chips, tortilla chips, sandwich meats, steak sauces, salad dressings, soft drinks, and so on. Monosodium glutamate (MSG), baking powder, baking soda, and many medications such as antacids also contain a lot of sodium.

The key to avoiding sodium is to learn to enjoy the unsalted tastes of food. Fortunately, the less salt you eat, the less you crave it. Having just spent three months exploring whole foods, you are well on the way to a low salt diet. Continue the good work by cooking with little or no salt. Take the salt shaker off the table and put it where it's an effort to get up and get it.

Read food labels carefully and pass up the items that list salt or sodium early in the list of ingredients. Cut way back on pickled vegetables and cured meats like ham and salami. Limit your intake of salted nuts, popcorn, pretzels, and the like. Many cheeses are high in salt also, so eat them in very small portions.

As before, take your time and spend three months "desalting" your diet before going on to the next step. When you visualize or do relaxation exercises, see yourself enjoying the natural, unsalted tastes of food.

### Reduce Caffeine

Caffeine is present in coffee, black and green tea, and colas. It's not fattening in itself. In fact, it depresses appetite a little, so avoiding caffeine is not so much a weight control issue as a health issue.

A pharmacologist friend of mine tells me that if caffeine were newly discovered today, it would have trouble passing the FDA safety tests for new drugs, and it would certainly be available only by prescription. Caffeine is a *powerful* stimulant that affects your entire body for hours after you injest it. It is addictive, producing cravings for more and withdrawal symptoms such as headaches when you stop taking it.

Caffeine also depletes your system of the B vitamins, which you need to fight stress.

If you can't cut out caffeine completely, try to get down to either one cup of coffee, two cups of tea, or two colas a day. Try decaffeinated versions of these drinks. For the next three months, use your relaxation and visualization exercises to remind yourself that "I don't need a jolt of caffeine to function. I'm alert and healthy on my own." Picture yourself enjoying herbal tea or orange juice with your nutritious breakfast.

### Take Supplements

Of course, you can implement this step at any time. The sooner the better. It's at the end of the chapter because the best source of vitamins and minerals is food—the kind of nutritious foods you have been spending months learning to love.

While you're in the health food store looking for alternative foods, spend some time in the supplement section. Collect some information and plan a reasonable program of supplementation for yourself.

## Special Considerations

If you've been adding up all the foregoing "three month plans," you've realized that I'm suggesting a *two-year* program here. That's a long time. But it's naive to think that you can permanently change the eating habits of a lifetime in any shorter period.

Some people have special nutritional needs: pregnant women, nursing mothers, diabetics, and those with numerous food allergies. If you fall into these categories, consult a doctor, counselor, support group or some other source of extra information and guidance. Make sure the person you select is in accord with your desire to achieve long-term weight control through gradual changes to your diet. Don't start fooling with your diet in any radical way until you understand your personal situation and needs.

Don't get carried away in your search for good nutrition. I once knew a happy, heedless girl, more than a little plump but unconcerned about it. She ate whatever she felt like: waffles for breakfast, burgers and fries for lunch, cheese and crackers and ice cream with chocolate sauce for dinner.

Then some well-meaning guidance counselor told her that she should become a hospital dietician. She started taking nutrition classes and changing her diet. She learned that the waffles had too much sugar, the burgers too much salt, and the cheese and ice cream too much fat. So she cut them out in favor of eggs and bacon, tuna sandwiches, and steak. Then she found out the eggs were loaded with cholesterol, the bacon had nitrites, the tuna was full of mercury, and the steak laced with hormones. So she switched to fresh fruit, spinach salad, and poached fish. But she learned subsequently that the fruit was contaminated with pesticides, the spinach contained high levels of a naturally occuring carcinogen, and that the fish was an endangered species.

The last time I saw my friend she was surviving on nothing but organic brown rice and free range turkey breast boiled in distilled water. And she was starting to have doubts about the turkey.

All right, this is a little exaggerated. But the point is that there is no single, perfect food or even a single, perfectly balanced diet that you can follow. You can find something wrong with every food.

# 6

# Increase Activity

I call this chapter "Increase Activity" instead of "Excercise More" because I want to avoid the usual connotations of exercise. I don't want you to automatically think of gyms, reducing salons, or Jazzercise®—or any other setting where exercise can become a grim, regimented program of hard work. This is not a chapter about doing the Jane Fonda workout on your living room rug every morning or running through the Canadian Airforce Exercises religiously.

Increasing activity can mean just walking more often instead of driving your car, or using a spade insead of a rototiller. It's a lifestyle change, not a temporary program that you abandon after you've lost weight.

## Proper Goals

**Fun.** However you increase your activity, it has to be fun. Otherwise, you won't make it part of a new lifestyle. Buying a bike and riding it to work and on local errands is a great way to increase your activity.

But if it isn't fun for you, save your money. After the first few days, the bike will just gather dust in the basement. Find something that you genuinely enjoy, something that you look forward to from day to day.

**A more instrumental view of your body.** Remember, your body is an instrument for doing things, not just an ornament to look at. The goal of increasing your activity is not to get slimmer and look good. It is to *become a better instrument*, to be able to do more things and enjoy the capabilities of your body. Doing six jillion leg lifts a week to get firmer thighs is silly and hard to keep doing week after week. But walking up to the park to see the sunset after dinner each evening is something you can make an enjoyable part of your life. It's really *doing* something. You can stick with it and, by the way, have firm thighs as well.

**Fitness and health.** Again, forget about your thighs or your waist measurement. Concentrate on the advantages of a fit, healthy body. When you're fit, you notice three things: (1) You're more flexible, able to pick up a penny off the floor without debating about it for five minutes or groaning like a rusty gate. (2) You are stronger, able to hold two really heavy grocery bags in your arms and unlock the front door at the same time. (3) You have better endurance, capable of shoveling snow off the whole front walk without resting or climbing three flights of stairs without huffing and puffing.

You'll get further health benefits when your increased activity reaches aerobic levels—when you keep your heart beating fast for twenty minutes or more at a stretch. This has a "training effect" on your heart muscle, making it stronger. Your circulation will improve and you' ll stand less chance of high blood pressure or arteriosclerosis.

**Physical well being.** Increasing your activity will make you feel better physically. Your body craves excercise the way it craves food. You share with your primitive hunter-gatherer ancestors a body that is designed for walking or running nearly all day long. Only 25 percent of Americans are sufficiently active.

Increased activity fights chronic fatigue and insomnia better than coffee and sleeping pills. Immediately after some vigorous activity like taking a walk, you'll feel energized and alert. Later, you'll be able to sleep better.

**Fight depression.** Exercise cheers you up. Beyond the obvious explanation that you feel good because you've done something good for yourself, there seems to be a chemical connection between exercise and moods. Fifteen to twenty minutes of vigourous exertion releases natural chemicals called catecholamines into your bloodstream and endorphins into your brain. Depressed people are often deficient in catecholamines, and endorphins are your body's natural pain killers and mood elevators.

**Stress reduction.** The connection here is simple. Stress is defined as the condition of being in the fight-or-flight state of arousal, in which your body is prepared to fight or flee from some perceived threat. By jogging, swatting a tennis ball, or mowing the lawn, you reduce your arousal level in the most natural way, through physical exertion.

**Mental alertness.** Your mind is connected to and affected by your body in a thousand ways. When you're active, your improved physical tone translates directly into mental muscle. You think faster, see more clearly, remember better, converse more witti-ly, feel more curious about things, solve problems more creatively, and in general feel more interested in and enthusiastic about life.

**Love and appreciation for your body.**  If you're like most chronic dieters, you often feel hateful or resentful about your body. Increasing your activity and thus your fitness level will make it easier for you to love your body and appreciate what it can do for you. You may eventually find yourself having thoughts like "I'll give my body a special treat and go swimming."

**Companionship.**  If you choose group or team activities like volleyball, a bird watching club, or an aerobic dance class, companionship can be a valuable bonus. You can meet interesting people and even make new friends.

## Improper Goals

You're doomed from the start if you set out to "get more exercise" for many of the usual reasons shared by chronic dieters.

Don't excercise because you want to lower your setpoint weight. That's no fun and you won't stick to it.

Don't exercise to lose weight. As soon as you lose a little, you'll revert to your previous slothful exist-ence and gain more weight back.

Don't excercise to be beautiful or handsome. As soon as you slim down or put on a little muscle, you'll probably slack off and end up back where you started or worse.

Don't exercise to be "good." Increasing your activity will only work if you find something you like to do, not something you should do.

Don't exercise to prove your worthiness. You're already worthy—you don't have to prove it.

All these goals are improper in that they are bad for you emotionally. They set you up for disappointment and guilt.

## How Exercise Affects Weight

If you go on a diet and just sit around, you'll lose weight. But for every three pounds of fat you lose, you'll also lose about a pound of muscle. You'll end up thin but weak. On the other hand, if you go on the same diet while getting plenty of exercise, you'll not only lose weight faster, you'll also lose much more fat than muscle—about 20 pounds of fat for every pound of muscle lost. You'll end up thinner but not weaker.

Common sense offers a plausible explanation: while you're excercising, you are not only maintaining muscle tone and mass, you're also raising your metabolism so that you burn up extra calories to speed weight loss.

But it's actually a little more complicated than that.

Increased activity affects weight in a much more profound way than just burning up calories while you're excercising. Actually, you don't burn up all that many calories during vigorous exercise. The number of calories you burn while jogging or biking for twenty minutes is relatively insignificant compared to the number of calories you consume in a day.

The big difference comes from the fact that regular exercise increases your *basal* metaboism rate—the rate at which you burn up calories *when you're at rest*. That adds up to a very significant number of calories indeed.

So walking to work not only keeps you fit and burns up extra calories, it also keeps working while you're sitting at your desk. Playing tennis on Saturday morning helps keep you slim during Sunday brunch.

If you stay active and eat spontaneously without dieting, you may notice that you look and feel thinner, although you weigh about the same. That's because you've lost fat but gained muscle, which is relatively heavier and denser than fat. Judge your results by how you feel, not by how much you weigh.

## Traditional Exercise

When looking to increase your activity, at least consider traditional exercise. You might just like it. The first distinction that is usually made concerning formal, traditional exercise is whether it is aerobic or low-intensity.

### Aerobic Versus Low Intensity Exercise

Aerobic exercise involves sustained, rhythmic activity of large muscle groups—running, jogging, fast walking, swimming, cycling, and dancing. Aerobic exercise uses up lots of oxygen, increases your heart rate, your heart's stroke volume, your breathing rate, and the degree of relaxation of your small blood vessels. All of this has a "training effect" on your heart and circulation system. Over time, your heart muscle actually gets stronger and your stamina increases so that it's easier to do aerobic exercise. To achieve this training effect, you need to get your heart rate elevated and keep it there for at least twenty minutes, three times a week.

If you don't exercise much now, you should start with low-intensity exercise and save the aerobic kind for later. Low-intensity exercise includes slow walking, house cleaning, calisthenics, weight lifting, isometrics, bowling, and so on. Almost any physical activity can count as low-intensity exercise. It builds strength, flexibility, and joint mobility, but doesn't have a training effect on your heart because it's not vigorous or prolonged enough.

For weight control, either kind of exercise is OK, although aerobic exercise is probably better in terms of how fast it burns calories and raises your basal metabolism. But again, the key is not which kind of exercise is best. The key is which do you prefer? Try an aerobic dance class, weight lifting, swimming, team sports, or whatever turns you on. But don't make your choice based on what taxes your body the most or the "best." Find out what you like to do, then do more of it.

You probably get more low-intensity exercise than you realize. You can find out by wearing a pedometer for a week. A pedometer is a little instrument you can get a a sporting goods store. You clip it onto your belt and adjust it for the length of your stride. The pedometer counts your steps and translates them into miles. If you walk less than two and a half miles a day, you are pretty sedentary and should start increasing your activity slowly, with low-intensity exercises like walking or golf.

### Avoid Exercise Programs That Stress Weight Loss

Don't join a gym, aerobics dance class, yoga group, or other program where the focus is on weight loss. You know the kind of group I mean, where the leader is always saying things like "This one is great for taking inches off your hips." Remember that your goal is to change your lifestyle and enjoy being active—not to worry about weight or inches.

### Avoid Injury

You hear this whenever you hear about exercise, but it bears repeating. When you're not used to vigorous exercise, it's easy to injure yourself by starting too fast. Be sure to warm up completely before exercise, and cool down slowly afterward. Don't overdo it at first. Make sure you get good instruction. Invest in the right equipment, especially shoes. Skip your exercise when you're ill or very tired. Don't exercise after a heavy meal. Don't smoke after exercising. Keep it fun and keep it safe.

## Increased Activity

This is where it's really at. Face it, if tennis or jogging were really your thing, you'd be doing them already. If you're past your teens or early twenties and are not a committed spare time athlete, it's not terribly likely that you will suddenly become one.

Much more likely is a gradual, subtle change to a more active lifestyle, one that involves a little more walking and a little less riding, a little more stair climbing and a little less elevatoring, a little more gardening and a little less TV watching.

Increasing your activity level in general is easier because it isn't dependent on a team, a teacher, special equipment, a particular time of day, good weather, and so on. It involves a change in lifestyle, not a set of new skills and commitments. By making small changes to daily habits you already have, you can gradually change from a sedentary to an active person.

### Some Suggestions

Here are just a few examples of how you can inject activity into your everday life. Try these suggestions to get started. Soon you will start thinking of your body as an instrument to be used, and other opportuniies for enjoyable activity will become obvious to you.

Park your car in the farthest part of the parking lot instead of cruising around looking for the closest possible parking space.

Take the stairs instead of the elevator.

Use a hoe instead of the weed whacker, a push mower instead of the power mower, a handsaw instead of the power saw, a whisk instead of the food processor or mixer, and so on.

Do your own chores and errands instead of having your kids or spouse do them for you.

Go out to get a newspaper or a pizza instead of having them delivered.

Ride a bike or walk to work or school instead of driving or taking the bus. If you live too far away to pedal or walk the whole way, arrange to be dropped off a few blocks short of your destination and walk part of the way.

Clean your own house, wash your own car, or paint your own garage, rather than pay others to do these jobs for you.

Rearrange your house so that there is only one clock, one phone, one place for pencils and paper. This will force you to get up and move when you want to see what time it is, answer the phone, write a list, and so on.

Plant and care for a garden.

Disconnect your automatic garage door opener so that you'll have to get out of the car and physically raise the door.

Plan activities like hiking, bird watching, or visiting museums that require you to be up on your feet, rather than spending all your leisure time watching TV, going to movies, or riding around in a car.

Instead of automatically reaching for the TV controls when you want to be diverted, consider horsing around with the kids, baking bread, or walking the dog.

When you do sit around to relax, keep the snacks across the room—not so you'll eat less, but to make yourself get up to fetch them.

Deliberately put things you need frequently in the attic, basement, garage, or on high shelves, so that you'll have to expend some effort to get them.

Put on some music and just dance around the room for no reason.

Hide the TV remote control so you'll have to get up to change channels.

Volunteer to walk door-to-door for your favorite candidate or cause.

Join a local search-and-rescue team to get yourself out in the country on a regular basis.

You can probably see a pattern here. The key to increasing activity is to reverse the trend of our service-oriented, labor-saving lifestyle. It may seem at first that you will be disorganizing your life and exhausting yourself. But you may be surprised. Most sedentary people find that when they start to do more, the result is a net increase in their energy level, so that they feel less tired and more alive.

## Exercises

These exercises aren't situps or chinups. They are pen and paper exercises or experimental adjustments to your lifestyle to help you see what forms of increased activity will work best for you.

### Daily Diary

Keep track of your opportunities to be active and what you typically do about them. Follow the format used in the example below, noting the time, the possible activity, and the thoughts you have regarding doing or not doing the activity.

| Time | Possible Activity | Reason to do it or not |
|------|-------------------|------------------------|
| 7:00 | Walk dog | Running late, just let him out in the yard |
| 8:00 | Walk David to nursery school | Running late, drive him |
| 10:00 | Pick apples for applesauce | Too much trouble, I'll just buy some applesauce |
| 11:30 | Carry groceries to car | OK, it doesn't take any more time. |
| 2:00 | Walk David back from nursery school | Do it, plenty of time now |

| | | |
|---|---|---|
| 3:30 | Walk dog | Do it with son |
| 5:00 | Play puppet show with David | Too busy getting dinner ready, have him watch Sesame Street |
| 5:15 | Walk dog | Oh all right, it'll be fun |
| 7:00 | Go for walk after dinner | OK, let's go. It's more fun to exercise together. |
| 7:45 | Pick apples for sauce | A bonus—after the walk everybody pitched in to help |

In this example, a busy mother of a preschool child finds several opportunities to increase her activity. The pattern that develops over a few days of diary keeping is this: she tends to be rushed and busy in the mornings, so that she'll have to wake everyone up a little earlier and get them more organized if she wants time to walk her son to nursery school. She does best with small, spur- of-the-moment decisions like parking the car in a remote corner of the supermarket parking lot, carrying her groceries instead of wheeling them back to the car in a cart, lugging small rugs outside and shaking them instead of vacuuming them in place, spading her flower beds by hand instead of asking her neighbor to rototill, and so on. Her most enjoyable activities are playing with her son and taking walks with her whole family. As with the apples that finally got picked, she found that one activity led to another, and that, up to a point, increasing her energy expenditures actually increased her available energy.

When you keep your own diary, attune your mind to opportunities for increased activity. This doesn't mean that you have to engage in every activity you think of. Look for patterns that show what kinds of exercise you gravitate toward, what you shun like the plague, which times of day or circumstances make a difference for you, and so on.

Don't feel guilty about the activities you habitually avoid. Your reasons for not increasing your activity level are powerful—they have been keeping you from fulfilling a strong basic need for a long time. To change your behavior patterns, you will have to slowly and methodically refute your reasons for not exercising.

Here are some examples of reasons why people don't exercise and the refutations that have helped them overcome their old reasons. See if any of this mental self-talk sounds familiar.

| Reasons not to exercise | Refutations |
| --- | --- |
| I'm running late. | I can get up as soon as the alarm rings |
| I'm too old for this. | All ages need exercise. This is how I'll stay young for my age. |
| I'll have a heart attack. | I can get a checkup and find out. I can start slowly. |
| My schedule's already too full. | Exercise will make it seem like I have more time, not less. |
| It's no use, it's a drop in the bucket. | Every motion helps raise my metabolism and burn fat. |

On a separate piece of paper, write down your own recurrent reasons for not exercising. Then compose your own refutations. Try to make your arguments for exercising short and posiitve. Use them as affirmations that you say to yourself every time you encounter a chance to increase your activity. As you slowly change your thinking, your activity level will increase. It won't happen overnight or in a perfectly regular course. You can expect some setbacks and relapses of "sedentarianism." Be patient. Over time, you can change the habits of a lifetime.

### Trial Periods

Set up trial periods of one or two weeks. Choose one traditional kind of exercise such as jogging or Jazzercise® and try it for a week or two. During the same period, try a nontraditional form of increased activity such as nature walks or hand sanding instead of using a power sander. Work your way through as many possible sports and activities as you can think of or are available to you. Try each for a week or two, then drop it and go on to another. In a few months you will have quite a large selection of possibilities to choose from. You'll know what you like and what doesn't fit your style and capabilities. Go back and incorporate your favorites into your lifestyle.

## Special Considerations

### Start slowly

If you've been inactive, suddenly starting a vigorous exercise program could bring on a heart attack or severe muscle strain. See a doctor before starting to excercise if you are over thirty and overweight, if you are a smoker, if you have high blood pressure, if you have arterial narrowing, or if you have a high blood cholesterol level. If you aren't sure about your condition, see a doctor anyway. Your doctor may recommend a stress electrocardiogram if you're over forty.

### *For Women Who Have Never Exerted Themselves*

Our culture doesn't encourage women to exercise. Many myths and misconceptions have grown up around the subject of women and exercise. Here are the facts: it's OK for women to sweat. Women can exercise just as much as men. Even during menstrual periods, women's reproductive organs are better protected than men's. Women who exercise regularly have fewer complications during pregnancy, less cramping during periods, and an easier time of it during menopause. Women can and should exercise after childbirth. Weight lifting and other, similar activities will not give women bulging muscles, just stronger ones.

If you are a woman and seem too tired after exercise, you may have an iron deficiency. Try eating iron rich foods or taking an iron supplement.

# 7

# Stick to It

There must be some area of your life that is not a problem for you. Perhaps you make friends easily and almost never have the feeling that nobody cares about you. Or maybe you're mechanically inclined and seldom feel intimidated by things like cars and washing machines that break down. Or perhaps you have a green thumb and keeping your garden and landscaping in order is a joy rather than a chore for you.

In what activity are you more competent that the average person? What skill do you have that often puts you a step ahead of the crowd? What character trait do you have that makes a particular aspect of life easier for you than for others? It might be something very simple like a firm sense of direction that won't let you get lost, or a facility with math that keeps your checkbook always balanced, or a love of handicrafts that fills your empty hours. The list could go on and on.

Some people seem to be born with an ability to handle food and weight effortlessly. That's the area of life in which they naturally excel. They never give a thought to what they eat, they don't worry about what they weigh, and they look fine without ever dieting or making an effort to excercise.

If you stick with the previous six steps of this book, that's the kind of person you can become. You actually can change your lifestyle and thereby change yourself "for good."

This chapter will show you how to stick with your program of lifetime weight control by covering six important topics:

1. What it means to change your lifestyle
2. Using visualization and affirmations to reinforce change
3. Handling setbacks
4. Responding to crticism
5. Coping with holidays and parties
6. Cognitive techniques for rewarding yourself and changing stubborn habits

## Choose a Lifestyle, Not a Weight

A lifestyle is a collection of habits and attitudes that *come naturally*, that you adhere to because it's easy and you want to, not because you think you should. This where traditional diets go wrong. They have you choose a weight, then design a lifestyle of eating and exercising to reach that target weight. The lifestyle is unnatural to you and very unpleasant, so as soon as you reach the target weight, you revert to your old, natural, comfortable lifestyle and gain the weight back.

The secret to lifetime weight control is to choose a lifestyle first and seek it, accepting the weight that results. Choosing and seeking a lifestyle means that you gradually acquire habits of eating and exercise that please you, that you can live with day in and day out. You gradually form attitudes about food, exercise, and weight that make sense to you. You gradually adopt attitudes about yourself and others that allow you to be content and happy.

From this new lifestyle—this new collection of habits and attitudes—a particular setpoint weight range will result. You'll be able to stay in this setpoint range effortlessly, because it comes naturally from the kinds and amounts of eating and excercise that you can maintain effortlessly.

If you pursue a lifestyle that includes plenty of exercise, nutritious food, home-cooked meals, low stress levels, satisfying emotional relationships, and so on, you will probably settle into the lowest setpoint range possible for you. That would be easy to accept.

On the other hand, if you decide that a faster-paced life is more important to you, with little exercise, more junk food, more eating out, higher stress, less time for personal relationships, and so on—then you will probably settle into a higher setpoint weight range. And that will be harder to accept.

But note that *either is acceptable.* There's nothing morally wrong or medically dangerous about being a little heavier. It's all in your mind: if you can accept the weight range that results from your chosen lifestyle, you have no weight problem and have achieved lifetime weight control. This viewpoint is not glib doublethink; it's simply, literally true.

To sum up:  pursue a lifestyle, not a weight. Make sure the lifestyle includes the amounts and kinds of eating and exercise that please you. Then accept the setpoint weight range that results. The key to making weight control work over a lifetime is the acceptance, not the weight range.

## Visualization and Affirmations

"But how do I pursue a new lifestyle when I'm stuck in the old one?" Visualization and affirmations can help a lot.

Visualization helps you create a new image of yourself as a healthy, contented person, living a full and satisfying life at a reasonable setpoint weight, whatever that weight is. You reinforce this image by visualizing it daily, fleshing it out. Affirmations help remind you of your new self-image and of specific behaviors that you are trying to make into habits. As time goes by, you act more and more out of your new self-image, and less and less out of your old image of yourself as an unhappy, fat person.

### Visualizations

The visualization that follows is adapted from my book, *Visualization for Change*. It follows the course of an ideal day in your life. Since it is a too long to remember, you should tape-record the material and play the tape during your first few visualization sessions. When you're familiar with the material, start doing shorter segments from memory each day. For example, you might visualize the restaurant scenes before you go out to eat, or the breakfast scene before you go to sleep at night. Revise this visualization with details from your own life. Make it as true to your own life and as accurate as you can.

The best time to use visualization is when you are naturally relaxed. Just before falling asleep at night and before getting out of bed in the morning are good times.

The rules for visualization are simple: lie down, close your eyes, relax, and form mental sense impressions of the way you'd like to be. Try it right now.

Lie down on your back on a rug, bed, or couch. Uncross your legs and put your hands at your side or rest them lightly on your chest. Get completely comfortable.

Close your eyes and take a slow, deep breath. Continue to breathe slowly and deeply. This kind of breathing naturally relaxes your body.

Visualization works best when your body is relaxed. Let your attention wander over your body: your feet, legs, trunk, arms, neck, and head. Wherever you feel a little muscular tension or soreness, try to relax the muscles in that area. It will help to flex the muscles first, then let them go slack. For example, if your neck is tight and stiff, try shrugging your shoulders up for a moment and tensing your neck muscles. Then let your neck relax and elongate. Do this tensing and relaxing of any other part of your body that feels tight. Feel the slow tide of relaxation that flows over your body.

Now, with your eyes still closed, imagine that you are waking up in the morning. Drift from vague dreams to an awareness that it's morning and time to get up. Feel the weight and warmth of the covers. Imagine rubbing your eyes, opening them, and seeing your bedroom. Look at the clock and see what time it is. Stretch and yawn. Get out of bed. Go to the bathroom to take a shower or bath. You feel rested, wide awake, light, and healthy. You're glad to be alive and feel good in your body.

In the bath or shower, run your hands over your body as you wash. Notice that your skin is smooth and healthy looking. Note that your body seems firmer and leaner than usual. If any negative thoughts about your body come to mind, say to yourself, "Stop! I love my body just the way it is." Get out of the bath and look at yourself in the steamy bathroom mirror. Write with your finger on the mirror: "I love you." Really feel the slick, cool mirror and the muscles of your arm and hand moving as you write. See your face becoming clearer as you wipe the condensation away.

Now get dressed. Put on some new, attractive clothes that are exactly the right size for your body just as it is—not the size you *wish* you could wear. Feel how soft and luxurious the fabric feels on your clean, firm skin. Smell that "department store" smell that new clothes have. Look at yourself in a full-length mirror and notice how good you look in clothes that are the right size and don't pinch and squeeze you. Really enjoy the loose, free feel of clothes that fit.

Go into the kitchen and prepare some breakfast. Have some fruit, some cereal, whole grain toast, juice, or some other light, nutritious food. Take your time and enjoy. Savor your food and be sure to eat enough. Tell yourself, "I love food. Food is my friend. I eat what I want and need to stay healthy, active, and feeling good."

Walk out your front door with a spring in your step. Feel rested, satisfied, full of pep. Swing your arms and shoulders and hips a little more than usual, enjoying the sheer pleasure of moving in your healthy, well-nourished body.

Go to work, to school, or somewhere else where you have something to do that involves other people. Look at the other people and notice that they are all human beings, whether fat or skinny or "just right." All have needs and desires and dignity. Expand your standards until everybody looks "just right," just human.

Imagine that you are doing your work or going to classes. Allow yourself to feel different emotions. First, feel bored. Imagine that you have no interest in anything, that you are at loose ends. Allow the thought to enter your mind: "I could get something to eat." But instead, see yourself get up and go for a walk. Get some exercise and fresh air. Feel a renewed interest in your job or studies. Tell yourself, "I have many interesting things to do. I'm actually much too busy to think about food."

Now feel anxious. Feel like someone is going to criticize you or test you on something you don't know well. Allow yourself to think about food as a way to reduce the anxiety. But instead of heading for the cafeteria, the cafe, or the refrigerator, see yourself going into a quiet place and doing some deep, slow breathing to calm down. Feel your anxiety level decreasing. Tell yourself, "I'm a worthwhile person. I always do my best. If I make a mistake, I forgive myself. If I do well, I congratulate myself."

Next feel depressed. Let yourself slide way down. Nothing is worth bothering with. There is no hope. As the thought of food enters your mind, shout, "No! Eating will just make things worse. I can go jogging or swimming. I can take a brisk walk or do some aerobics. After all, I'm in control of my life. I can solve my problems step by step."

Feel angry. Imagine experiencing some insult or slight or unfairness. But pretend that it seems too dangerous to show your anger. Stifle it. Think of some way to smother your anger or console yourself, like eating some ice cream. But instead of heading for the freezer, dial the phone and call up a friend or relative. Tell that person about your anger. Say, "I just had to talk to somebody about this. I'm so angry." Feel your anger, and your false hunger, fading away as you tell your story. Think to yourself, "I alone am responsible for my life and my feelings. I can acknowledge my anger. I can work through it. I can avoid getting angry next time. I can forgive others and myself."

Finally, feel stressed out. Imagine that there are a million deadlines and demands on your time. Let the pressure build. Feel the intense craving to take a break for some coffee and a donut. But instead, see yourself taking a deep breath and letting it out slowly. Watch your eyes close. Feel the deep, slow breathing as it calms your body and washes away the feeling of pressure. Feel your muscles unclench as you count your slow breaths and relax. See yourself opening your eyes and calmly beginning to organize your time, all thoughts of a donut break vanished. Say the affirmations: "I am a grownup person, intelligent and sensitive. I seldom think about food between meals."

Now you notice that it's time to go to lunch. Walk to a favorite restaurant. On the way, look at your reflection in the shop windows. Just for fun, imagine that you have suddenly become skinny as a stick. See yourself as a "ninety-pound weakling." Does it scare you? Do you feel suddenly unprotected, like you've lost your armor against the world? Repeat to yourself, "I can weigh less and still be strong. I can protect myself. I can be safe without my armor of fat."

Resume your normal shape and go on to the restaurant. Go inside and notice the sights, sounds, and smells. Take a moment to concentrate on the details of the scene. Scan your body again and relax any muscles that have become tight.

Open the menu. As you scan the choices, look for what you really want to eat. Tell yourself, "I trust my body. It knows what I need." See yourself ordering exactly what you want, not what you think is low-calorie or proper. If you want fries and a milkshake, go ahead. If you want a cocktail, some wine or beer, or some coffee, go ahead and order it. If you have a problem moderating your intake of these things, see yourself declining them or having just one serving.

When your lunch comes, enjoy it. Taste and smell your food. Feel its temperature and texture in your mouth. Gradually feel fuller and fuller, less and less hungry. When you're full, put your fork down and push your plate away. Talk to your companion if you have one, or imagine reading a good book until the check comes. Tell yourself, "I always know the instant I'm full. I'd rather leave food on the plate that eat more than I want and feel stuffed."

On the way out of the restaurant with some change in your hand, pass an old fashioned pay scale. Put your change in your pocket or purse and pass the scale by. Tell yourself that you're not interested in how much you weigh. How you feel is more important.

Take a walk around town. Enjoy your full but not stuffed feeling. Notice the weather, the traffic, the trees and buildings. Pass by a theater that is showing an R-rated movie. Look at the poster and think about sex. If it makes you nervous, tell yourself, "I accept my own sexuality. I can handle sexual advances. As I get firmer and more attractive, I also get more confident. I'm becoming more assertive every day."

Walk past a park with tennis courts. Pause and watch some good players volleying. As you think about sports and competition, tell yourself, "I choose when and where I want to compete. I weigh what I have chosen to weigh. I can choose to weigh more or less. I am in control of my life."

Go home and sit there for a while. Spend some time by yourself until you start to feel a little lonely. Nobody's around, you're all by yourself and beginning to feel a little sorry for yourself. Maybe you should go get a little treat to make yourself feel better. But no. Instead, you call up a friend. Imagine that your friend cheers you up and invites you to come over after dinner.

Go out for a while and get some exercise. Take a walk, go jogging or cycling, go to the gym or go swimming, take an aerobics class, or whatever. See yourself as enjoying the exercise for its own sake, not because it's part of a weight-loss program. Tell yourself, "I exercise regularly because I love it."

Turn on the TV or page through a magazine, looking at the skinny people in the ads. Shake your head in disbelief and amusement. Tell yourself, "Those are just teenagers, dressed up to look like adults. The older ones either have unusually low setpoint weights or they must suffer constantly to be that slim."

Fix a light, well-balanced dinner, something you really like. Take your time and enjoy it. The moment you feel full, get up and start clearing the table. Tell yourself, "I take care of myself. I eat plenty of good food and I'm happy at my setpoint weight."

Go over to your friend's house. Meet several of your friends there for an impromptu party. Have just one or two drinks, and maybe just a little of the abundant party food. Tell yourself, "At parties, I'd rather talk or dance than eat. I can have a good time without eating constantly."

Watch yourself at the party. See yourself as a little fitter, slightly lighter, moving gracefully, and smiling. Feel comfortable in your well-fitting clothes. Enjoy the feeling of health and vitality in your body. Love your body just the way it is. See your friends laughing and smiling while talking to you.

Look forward in time and see yourself at the same healthy setpoint weight year after year, feeling good, enjoying food, and not even thinking about weight control or dieting.

Now end this visualization by reminding yourself of your actual surroundings as you lie there. When you are ready, open your eyes and get up.

### Affirmations

In the visualization above, you were asked to tell yourself things like "I seldom think about food between meals" and "I take care of myself." These kinds of affirmations should be familiar to you after working through some of the exercises in the previous chapters. Affirmations are short, positive statements about yourself, designed to reinforce changes you are trying to make in your lifestyle. They are cast in the present tense, as if the desired change has already been accomplished.

Affirmations act like posthypnotic suggestions,

influencing your behavior and attitudes, giving you little shoves in the direction you want to go. They work best when you make up two or three at a time and repeat them to yourself throughout the day.

In making up affirmations about your new weight control lifestyle, be sure to follow these guidelines: keep affirmations short, keep them simple, and keep them postive. For example, don't say "I'm not obsessed with food." Research has shown that your subconscious mind doesn't understand negative words very well. It is likely to interpret this statement as "I'm obsessed with food," dropping out the "not."

Here are some examples of affirmations that have worked well for others:

- I am a grown-up person.
- I am intelligent and sensitive.
- I am in control of my life.
- I choose what I want.
- Only I am responsible for my life.
- I am a worthwhile person.
- When I do something good, I congratulate myself.
- When I make a mistake, I forgive myself.
- I make reasonable plans for the future.
- I ignore things in the future that are beyond my control.
- I enjoy food, but it is only moderately important to me.
- I eat just enough to stay healthy, active, and feeling good.
- I seldom think about food between meals.
- I always know the instant I'm full and stop eating then.

- I'd rather talk to a friend than eat.
- When I'm bored, I go for a walk instead of eating.
- I seldom weigh myself or think about my weight.

Notice that many of these affirmations deal with important issues that underlie weight control: self-esteem, responsibility, handling worry, and so on. Others are more specific to eating and weight. You should make up about a dozen affirmations of each kind for yourself. Put them in your own words for best results.

Use two or three of your affirmations frequently during the day. Say them silently to yourself, or out loud if possible. Write them down in the three-step technique described in the chapter on self-acceptance. This is a good way to not only impress an affirmation on your mind but also uncover and root out the negative remarks you may be making to yourself to undermine the effectiveness of an affirmation.

To stitch affirmations into the fabric of your daily life, try synchronizing them with routine daily acts. For example, every time you flush the toilet, say, "I seldom think about my weight." Every time you turn the ignition key in your car, think, "I am in control of my life." Each time you use the stapler or the copier or the hammer, tell yourself, "I take things one step at a time." When you reach for the salt shaker, remind yourself, "I always stop eating the instant I'm full."

Let your affirmations run through your mind when you're doing repetitive tasks. Rake leaves to the beat of "I can handle food in my life." Let the rhythm of the windshield wipers beat out "More rest, less food, more rest, less food." While painting your bedroom, focus on a different affirmation each time you replenish your roller or brush.

As suggested in earlier chapters, it's also a good idea to write your affirmations on three-by-five cards. Put the affirmation on one side and the negative thought or behavior it's designed to counter on the other side. Carry a couple of cards with you at all times. Pull them out whenever you have a moment and read the negative side first, then the positive side.

Write affirmations on Post-it® notes and stick them up wherever you will see them frequently:  on mirrors, on the refrigerator, on the TV, on the dashboard of your car, in your school binder or purse or briefcase or toolbox, on your typewriter, and so on. If you don't want these little ads for yourself tacked up all over where people can see them, use little colored dot stickers that you can get at stationery or toy stores. Let an orange dot on the bathroom mirror stand for "I eat only nutritious food." Put a purple dot on the telephone to remind yourself to "Keep moving, keep exercising."

Using visualization and affirmations this way is not a flakey, "new age" notion that some guru dreamed up in a crystal ball or translated from dolphin squeaks. Cognitive therapists have been using these techniques for years, giving them names like *covert modeling, systematic desensitization*, and *refuting irrational self-talk*. It comes down to the same simple ideas: visualize yourself accomplishing the things you desire and use short affirmations as reminders of the new attitudes and habits you are cultivating.

## Handling Setbacks

Setbacks are inevitable. Human willpower is not actually very powerful. Programs like Alcoholics Anonymous and Overeaters Anonymous recognize the weakness of willpower, and warn against depending on it.

Sheer will power will carry you for a matter of days or weeks. The seven steps outlined in this book will take you two or three years to make a natural part of your life. In that time, willpower alone will fail many times. You are bound to backslide. So the first step in handling setbacks is to realize that they are inevitable.

### Forgive Yourself

When you slip back into old, unwanted habits, your first inclination is probably self-criticism: "I'm eating too much junk, what a slob," "I'm so lazy, I haven't been swimming for two weeks," or "Why do I do what I don't want to do?"

When you start dumping on yourself, you scuttle your self-esteem and slide back into your former obsession with weight and dieting. You get depressed or anxious or angry. In this state, you're likely to lose even more ground.

Forgiving yourself is the answer. When setbacks happen, tell yourself, "Oh, here's one of those inevitable setbacks I read about, right on schedule." Take it as a sign that your lifetime weight control program is working as planned. Remind yourself that human progress is not a straight line affair—there must be valleys and plateaus in the climb to success.

If you find yourself wailing "But why do I always do what I don't want to do?" and you feel out of control, consider this: *you're always doing what seems best at the time.* You are in control whether it seems like it or not. In every situation, you consider your options and make a choice based on your awareness at the moment.

For example, Trudi would often have a milkshake and nothing else for lunch. She knew the shakes were full of fat and sugar and little else of nutritional value, so she decided to cut back. But even after she resolved to have a sandwich instead, she found herself ordering her favorite milkshake. She thought, "I'm weak, I'm out of control."

But she was actually in control, making choices all the time. She was choosing the pleasure of the milkshake over the nutrition of the sandwich, and choosing the security of an old ritual eating pattern over the insecurity of trying something new. In other words, Trudi ultimately found the milkshake more valuable for her than her new nutritional values.

These kinds of choices may not be wise ones, but they are genuine choices, not a "loss of control." You always choose what seems best for you at the moment, according to how reality looks to you and your values. If you want to change your habitual choices, you need to learn some nutritional facts so that you see reality more clearly and adopt new values. It's a learning process, a process you've initiated by reading this book.

### Practice Damage Control

The seven steps to lifetime weight control are like building blocks that make up a pyramid. The first step—not dieting any more—is the bottom layer. It's the foundation that supports the whole structure. The next step—self-acceptance—rests upon the first and in turn supports the third, and so on to the top of the pyramid.

Your pyramid will get jostled many times. The trick is to practice damage control by giving up the top of the pyramid first. When times get rough, abandon the seven steps in the reverse order that they are given in this book.

This is easy because it's the natural course of backsliding anyway. Exercise is usually the first to go. Then good nutrition. Then you start eating for company, for comfort, and so on, instead of satisfying those emotional needs directly. Then you lose consciousness of how and what and why you're eating. Finally, you stop accepting your weight, appearance, and behavior. You might even be shaken to the foundation and start dieting again.

But even if you do relapse all the way to your original chronic dieting behavior, you can practice damage control all the way. You can preserve some sense of control by noticing each step of the way and remaining conscious of the fact that you are making the choices that seem best at the time.

Acknowledge that you are giving up your physical activities in the interest of a busy schedule. Admit that you value your time more than exercise and are making that choice at this stage of your life. Resolve to get back in shape as soon as you have more time.

When the cheese puffs and candy bars start sneaking back into your diet, stay conscious of the fact that you know better. Don't condemn yourself. Eat well when you can get it together to do so, and try to keep your emotional life separate from your eating.

When you catch yourself eating to satisfy your need for love or security, at least congratulate yourself on remaining conscious of that fact.

When you find that you're looking critically in the mirror and running yourself down about your weight, remind yourself of your past successes with self-acceptance. Resolve to dig out your notebooks and go over your affirmations about acceptance.

**If you must diet**. If you backslide all the way and actively try to lose weight again, you can still practice damage control by chosing the *least harmful* means of weight loss. In order of preference, these are:

1. Exercise. Join an exercise group that stresses weight loss. Ignore what they say about dieting and just gets lots of vigorous exercise. This is good for your body and will help you lose weight without disrupting your eating patterns or plunging you into the ups and downs of chronic dieting again.

2. Consciousness raising. Join a support group that helps members explore cultural expectations, subconscious desires to be heavy, self-esteem, values clarification, weight as a feminist issue, and so on. Again, this will stimulate your mind, help with self-acceptance, and quite possibly result in some weight loss.

3. Programmed eating. This is the kind of diet where you follow a rigid menu for each meal, eating modest amounts of all kinds of nutritious food, with no substitutions allowed. Some of the newer group plans take this approach, providing all the food and group support as well. Choose a plan that lets you eat all you want of the approved menu, so that your body won't experience starvation and trap you in an

upward spiral of escalating setpoint weight. These plans can be expensive if you count the cost of the special food, but they work fairly well without disrupting your appetite and metabolism too much.

4. Permanent diet change. This is where you give yourself an ultimatum: "No more butter fat," "No more white flour," "No more refined sugar products," and so on. This kind of dieting has at least one thing going for it: as long as your ultimatums are based on good nutrition, the change will be good for your physical health. But "permanent" diet change usually doesn't last very long, since it typically arises out of a purely intellectual decision, not a gradual change of attitude and lifestyle. Permanent diet change relies too much on willpower and depriving yourself of foods you still enjoy. It can result in cravings and regaining lost weight (and then some) when your willpower gives out.

5. Slow traditional weight loss diet. This is where you count calories or eat controlled amounts of a nutritionally balanced menu. It's more damaging than the kind of permanent diet change described above. The only thing it has going for it is that it's slow—the slower the better. Weight comes off slowly, feelings of deprivation and cravings are milder than on crash diets, and after the diet weight is regained relatively slowly. Nevertheless, traditional weight loss diets are harmful to your body and your mental health.

6. Crash starvation or single-food diet. This is where you just starve, hardly eating anything but a little grapefruit, celery, liquid protein, or a very short list of low calorie foods. Starvation diets are hard on your body and your mind during the diet, and just

make you gain more weight back when you finally go off them. The starvation diet is the next-to-last choice, with nothing to recommend it except that there are no drugs involved.

7. Starvation diet with pills. Add powerful stimulant "diet pills" to the above and you have a sure recipe for disaster. Pray that your damage control procedures keep you from backsliding this far.

## Responding to Critics

In terms of your lifetime weight control program, there are only two kinds of people—those who support your efforts and those who don't.

### Getting Support

Lifetime weight control is very difficult without a minimum amount of support from family and friends. If you're having a hard time getting people to take you seriously, stop hassling you about your weight, and let you eat what you want, then go back to the end of the chapter on getting emotional needs met. Use the Support Agreement there to make one last attempt to get those around you to help, or at least stop hindering.

Asking someone to sign or even read a contract to support you may seem very contrived and embarrassing. But if you can bring yourself to do it, you will reap great benefits. If you just ask "Will you support me in this lifetime weight control thing?" people often tune you out. They can't agree until they know exactly what you mean by "support."

For example, going over the Support Agreement with your spouse can show that it's possible to help you without completely giving up his or her own beliefs or lifestyle. Read each item on the agreement together and cross out the efforts your spouse isn't willing to make. Circle the kinds of support your spouse is willing to give. Even if you your spouse agrees only to let you eat what you want, stifle critical comments, and not tempt you with junk foods, that will help a lot.

### Handling Unwelcome Criticism

You may still be left with a few people in your life who are just not going to be supportive. They may tease you, belittle your efforts, encourage you to try the latest diet, ask you why you don't diet, blame you for being out of shape, want you to dress or act differently, question your willpower, push food on you, and so on.

The first thing to do when you hear a critical remark is to keep quiet for a moment. Take a couple of seconds to recover from the natural shock of hearing someone's negative opinion of you. Tell yourself, "Others are entitled to their opinions. It doesn't mean they're right about me."

Then keep quiet some more. Stifle your automatic impulses to strike back, argue, or apologize. Recall this section of the book and use one of these assertive responses:

**Agreement (Yes, you're right.)** Nothing stops a critic like agreement. Your mom points out that you've been working on this lifetime weight control stuff for two months and you haven't lost any weight. It's true, so you just say, "Yep, that's right." And it stops there. Your husband complains that you've been serving some new kinds of vegetable dishes that you never used to cook, and you respond, "Yes, I have been trying a lot of different kinds of vegetables lately," and then keep quiet. Just being heard and acknowledged is enough for some critics. They won't start a fight unless you get defensive.

Don't use agreement unless what the critic says is actually true. If you consistently agree to false, negative statements about yourself, you'll damage your self-esteem.

**Partial agreement (Yes, you're right that...)** Sometimes you can stop a critic by agreeing with just one little part of what is said. For instance, your brother might say, "If I were you, I'd go on a crash diet and get down to my ideal weight, then go on a lifetime maintenance diet. You'd lose weight in a hurry, see some real results, and be way ahead of the game." You wouldn't agree with his entire proposal, but you could respond: "You're right, I would lose weight in a hurry." That part is true and hearing you admit it would probably shut him up, even though you didn't agree with all his ideas.

Again, don't agree even in part unless you actually can find something true to agree to.

**Explanation (No, you're wrong because...)** Then there are the important people with whom you have ongoing conversations about weight, whose support you hope to some day win, the ones you live with or see often, those who are very worried about your well being, and so on. They probably aren't quieted for long by token agreement.

The first few times you hear a critical point of view, you can explain. Tell your brother, "No, I'm not going on a crash diet first. I know from experience that I will be so miserable and crazy about food by the end of the diet that I will gain all the weight back again. I'll be further behind, not way ahead."

When your mother points out that you're still the same weight, you can say, "I appreciate your concern, but let me explain why I'm not worried myself: I've been reading and thinking a lot about weight control, and I'm following a very long-term plan now. Give me some time."

**Subject change (We'll never agree, so let's talk about ...)** With some people, your attempts at explanation won't quiet their criticism. They won't or can't accept new information that contradicts their predjudices. When they repeatedly take you to task about your weight or your program of lifetime weight control, change the subject gently but firmly: "You know, we've talked about this several times before, and I think I have a good idea of your feelings about this. I'd much rather talk to you about where you're going on vacation. Have you picked a hotel yet?"

Suggest a topic that you know the other person enjoys talking about. Plan in advance which questions you will ask to distract the other person and lure him or her onto another subject.

**Refusal (I won't discuss this with you.)** With really persistent people, you may have to be more direct: "Look, every time we talk about dieting and weight control I get upset. We go round and round with the same old arguments. The fact is, you'll never convince me I'm wrong, and I'll never convince you I'm right. I just don't want to talk about it anymore."

When the other person tries repeately to provoke you into a response, just keep refusing to talk about it like a broken record:

*Other:* But I just want to know what you think you're accomplishing.

*You:* I don't want to talk about it.
*Other:* I hate to see you deluding yourself.
*You:* I'm not going to talk about it.
*Other:* But you're not being reasonable.
*You:* It doesn't matter what you say, I don't want to talk about it.
*Other:* Well, OK then, be that way.

**Avoidance (Goodbye.)** The final resort is to leave or send the other person away. If partial agreement, explanations, changing the subject, and refusal to talk about it won't work, you have no choice but to avoid this person.

If your persistent critic is your spouse, someone you live with, a parent or other close relative whom you see often, or a close co-worker or friend whom you can't easily avoid, you have a serious problem. You should probably postpone working on lifetime weight control and work on changing or ending the relationship with the critic.

You may not have much success with weight control until a separation, divorce, move, new job, or couple's therapy removes you from constant criticism.

## Parties and Holidays

When you're on a strict diet, parties and holidays are big problems. When you're practicing lifetime weight control, the problem isn't so big. If you are eating more nutritous food and staying active 350 days of the year, it doesn't really matter much what you eat or how inactive you are for the other fifteen days surrounding Christmas, Hanukkah, New Year's, your birthday, and so on.

The first thing to do is give yourself some slack. Remember that you're interested in the long term, not how much pumpkin pie you eat today. Realize that there will be fatty and sugary foods around, no matter how you campaign for healthier fare. Count on there being more stress—the excitement of celebrating with loved ones, the horror of celebrating with loved ones, the misery of shattered expectations, and so on. Be ready for the inevitable tension and confusion. Don't add to it by beating yourself up about how much you eat.

Remember the emotional self-care plans you made in the chapter on satisfying emotional needs? You made up affirmation cards such as "When I'm bored I go to the library" and "When I feel lonely I go out for coffee with a friend." You can use the same technique to prepare for the situations that get you down at parties and holiday time. Make up cards and carry them around with you a few days before the upcoming events and during the festivities. Here are some examples.

- When I see the buffet, I look over each item before filling my plate.
- When others are eating, I don't automatically have to eat.
- When I eat Thanksgiving dinner, I take a tiny dab of each thing, then go back for seconds if I want.
- I can leave food on my plate at Grandma's house.
- When I have leftovers after the holidays, I pop them right into the freezer.
- When I eat sweets, I can stop after just one.
- When I go to parties, I eat a good meal before.

- When Christmas is at my house, I have a plan for each day.
- When I eat, I really notice what I'm eating and enjoy it.
- When I get nervous around Dad, I go into another room instead of eating.
- When I get unwanted food gifts, I open them right up, pass them around, and dump the leftovers as soon as I'm alone.
- When I get angry at my sisters, I go look at the photo album instead of snacking in the kitchen with Mom.
- When offered appetizers, I can say I'm saving room for dinner.
- When offered seconds, I can say I'm saving room for dessert.
- When offered dessert, I can say I'm waiting till later.
- When they start sitting around watching football, I can go jogging.
- When I start feeling left out, I think "I am a unique, valuable person just the way I am."
- When I start feeling impatient, I tell myself "They are doing the best they know how."
- I don't have to have a glass in my hand at every moment.
- I'll eat my veggies first, then anything I want.
- I'll be sure to take my vitamins.
- At parties, I'd rather dance and talk than eat.
- I'm ready to forgive myself for eating what looks good at the time.
- When I stuff myself I don't make it worse by blaming myself.

The key to surviving holidays and parties is to be prepared ahead of time. Know what you're going to do and what you're going to tell yourself. It will help a lot to do a long visualization in which you watch yourself coping successfully with all the temptations and problems that you expect to meet.

After the party or holiday meal, congratulate yourself on the parts that went well, and forgive yourself for the parts that didn't go so well. Make a note of what to do differently next time, then let go of the experience and don't dwell on it any longer.

## Cognitive Techniques for Change

### Rewards

From moment to moment, lifetime weight control involves lots of little decisions and actions such as glancing away from the magazine rack with its headlines about new miracle diets, making the extra effort to cook a vegetable to go with dinner, or choosing to walk to the drugstore instead of driving. These changes are hard to make at first, even though you know you will benefit from them eventually.

The way to turn these difficult changes into easy habits is to reward yourself. Each time you successfully perform some new behavior that you've been trying to make part of your life, consciously give yourself a treat.

Of course, I'm not talking about edible treats here. If you have been in the habit of rewarding yourself with food, that may be the only kind of treat you can easily think of. You need to expand your repertoire of pleasant rewards so that you can reward yourself whenever and wherever you are.

A reward can be an object, an action, a sound, a place, an experience, or even a thought. Anything that brings you a little pleasure and enjoyment qualifies as a reward. Here are some suggestions.

- Smell a flower.
- Take a nap.
- Go for a drive.
- Have a bubble bath.
- Hum a favorite tune.
- Get a new scarf.
- Stop off at the nursery.
- Sit down a minute and rub your feet.
- Get some flowers.
- Buy some new earrings.
- Listen to a favorite tape or record.
- Take a good stretch and yawn.
- Make a call to a special friend and chat.
- Leaf through a magazine.
- Watch a favorite TV program.
- Get a massage.
- Think about vacation.
- See yourself at the beach.
- Imagine playing violin in an orchestra.
- Imagine catching a big fish.
- Relive a pleasant memory.
- Visualize how fit and healthy you'll be.

Be sure to include pleasant mental images in your list of rewards. They can be entertained anywhere, no matter what else you're doing. That's important because rewards are most effective when they follow immediately after the behavior you're trying to encourage. As soon as you accomplish one of your desired actions, reward yourself with a quick mental sense impression: the feeling of your stronger muscles, the sound of your lover saying "I love you," an image of your child smiling, the feeling of warm sun on your skin, the taste of watermelon on the Fourth of July, and so on.

For big accomplishments, you might want more than a mental reward. If you can't immediately do anything for yourself, use a token reward. Put a penny in your shirt pocket or shopping bag to be "redeemed" later for a nap, a bath, or a game of bridge.

The flip side of reward is punishment. Some cognitive therapists suggest using aversive images as punishments for doing things you're trying not to do anymore. For example, when you start eating cookies in front of the television, you might try imagining someone you admire bawling you out.

Be careful if you try this technique. Don't use images of yourself as a fat person or other self-derogatory images that could undermine your self-esteem. If you have trouble with self-acceptance, the mental punishment approach can really backfire.

Whenever possible, it's better to figure out a new, positive action that you can take to replace the bad habit, and then reward yourself whenever you perform the alternative action. For example, you could plan to eat popcorn instead of cookies in front of TV, or do something to keep your hands busy such as crocheting a muffler or doing your nails. When you succeed, you should reward yourself with a romantic fantasy or by staying up to watch a special show.

Use different rewards for your different weight control goals. After a few weeks of rewarding a particular action it will become habitual and you will be able to do it without the reward. Then you can use that reward to reinforce another healthy habit.

### Breaking Stubborn Habits

This is a technique for breaking those habits that just seem to persist no matter how hard you try. It involves writing down exactly what you do, in as many tiny steps as possible. The idea is that any troublesome behavior is made up of a long string of actions or "decision points." You may feel like you just fall into or give into certain habits, but actually you perform a long series of actions that can be stopped at many points along the way.

Joe was a driving instructor who had a problem with eating ice cream after lunch. Almost every day he would have lunch at the same cafe. He'd have a sandwich and a glass of apple juice or some other reasonable choice. Then he would leave the cafe and go down to the corner ice cream parlor and have a hot caramel sundae and a cup of coffee. Even though he felt full after lunch and he knew he didn't need the sundae, he kept doing it.

Joe was pretty successful at his other weight control goals. He had stopped dieting, improved his nutrition in general, and was enjoying new activities like weight lifting and sailing. He was working on expressing his needs better in his relationship and rarely binged on beer and chips like he used to when he was anxious. But he couldn't stop his caramel sundae habit.

He tried inventing an alternative: going to the nearby park and reading the newspaper after lunch. And he planned to reward himself by scanning the

want ads and fantasizing about buying a used sail-
boat. But it didn't help. He rarely made it to the park.

Joe finally broke his habit by making this decision
checklist:

### Ice Cream Checklist

☐ 1. Finish last of apple juice and think how
good a sundae would taste (I could look forward to
the park).

☐ 2. Think of having some coffee with it (I could
plan where I'll sit in the park).

☐ 3. Get up and walk toward door (I could feel
in my pockets for change to buy a paper).

☐ 4. Walk out cafe door and turn left toward ice
cream parlor (I could turn right toward the park).

☐ 5. Pass the newstand (I could buy a paper and
turn back).

☐ 6. Push "walk" button to cross the street (I
could cross the other direction and double around to
the park).

☐ 7. Cross street (I could keep going straight and
go the other way to the park).

☐ 8. Open door to ice cream parlor (I could walk
past).

☐ 9. Enter parlor (I could open door and leave).

☐ 10. Sit down (I could still leave).

☐ 11. Order sundae and coffee (I could just have
coffee).

☐ 12. Wait for order (I could change to just a dish
of plain ice cream).

☐ 13. Pick up spoon when sundae comes (I could
just drink the coffee).

☐ 14. Take first bite (I could just eat a little and
leave the rest).

Joe made ten copies of this list and put them on the clipboard he usually carried around. While he was eating lunch each day in his favorite cafe, he put a fresh copy of the checklist on the clipboard at the side of his plate. His rule was that he was allowed to go for a sundae if he consciously made all fourteen decisions in sequence. To make sure he remained conscious of his actions, he read each item and checked it off before he did it.

Using the checklist slowed Joe down considerably. It made him think about what he was doing. It destroyed the usual momentum of habit that would propel him into the ice cream parlor. He had time to think of his alterntive behavior and the rewards of doing it, both short-term and long-term. He sometimes had the sundae anyway, but more and more often he decided to go to the park. Going to the park was just easier than checking off all those little boxes.

When you try this technique yourself, make sure you have at least a dozen steps. The more the better. As you use your checklist, you'll find that there are more decision points than you thought. Add them to the list until it's as long and complex as you can make it. Include at each step an alternative that will move you toward the replacement behavior you have planned.

# Other New Harbinger Self-Help Titles

*The Relaxation & Stress Reduction Workbook, 3rd Edition*, $13.95
*Leader's Guide to the Relaxation & Stress Reduction Workbook*, $14.95
*Beyond Grief: A Guide for Recovering from the Death of a Loved One*, $10.95
*Thoughts & Feelings: The Art of Cognitive Stress Intervention*, $12.95
*Messages: The Communication Skills Book*, $11.95
*The Divorce Book*, $10.95
*Hypnosis for Change: A Manual of Proven Techniques, 2nd Edition*, $11.95
*The Deadly Diet: Recovering from Anorexia & Bulimia*, $10.95
*Self-Esteem*, $11.95
*The Better Way to Drink*, $10.95
*Chronic Pain Control Workbook*, $12.50
*Rekindling Desire*, $10.95
*Life Without Fear: Anxiety and Its Cure*, $9.95
*Visualization for Change*, $11.95
*Guideposts to Meaning*, $10.95
*Controlling Stagefright*, $10.95
*Videotape: Clinical Hypnosis for Stress & Anxiety Reduction*, $24.95
*Starting Out Right: Essential Parenting Skills for Your Child's First Seven Years*, $12.95
*Big Kids: A Parent's Guide to Weight Control for Children*, $10.95
*Personal Peace: Transcending Your Interpersonal Limits*, $10.95
*My Parent's Keeper: Adult Children of the Emotionally Disturbed*, $11.95
*When Anger Hurts*, $11.95
*Free of the Shadows: Recovering from Sexual Violence*, $11.95
*Resolving Conflict With Others and Within Yourself*, $11.95
*Liftime Weight Control*, $10.95

Send a check or purchase order for the titles you want, plus $1.50 for shipping and handling, to:

New Harbinger Publications
Department B
5674 Shattuck Avenue
Oakland, CA 94609

Or write for a free catalog of all our quality self-help publications.